MW01394144

DATE DUE

J
615.78
DUR

DURHAM, MICHAEL
JUST THE FACTS
PAINKILLERS &
  TRANQUILIZERS

Just the Facts
Painkillers and Tranquilizers

Michael Durham

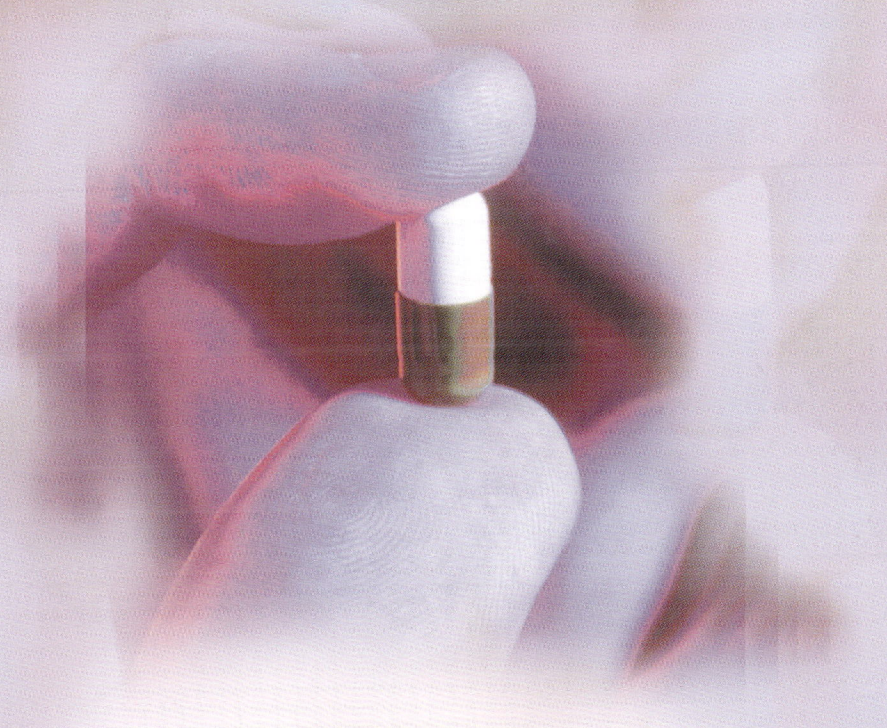

Heinemann Library
Chicago, Illinois

© 2003 Heinemann Library
a division of Reed Elsevier Inc.
Chicago, Illinois

Customer Service 888-454-2279
Visit our website at www.heinemannlibrary.com

All rights reserved. No part of this publication may be reproduced or transmitted in any form or by any means, electronic or mechanical, including photocopying, recording, taping, or any information storage and retrieval system, without permission in writing from the publisher.

Designed by Jane Hawkins
Originated by Ambassador Litho Ltd.
Printed and bound in China by South China Printing Company

07 06 05 04 03
10 9 8 7 6 5 4 3 2 1

Library of Congress Cataloging-in-Publication Data
Durham, Michael, 1952-
 Painkillers and tranquilizers / Michael Durham.
   p. cm. -- (Just the facts)
Summary: Offers a description of drugs used to treat pain, anxiety, and depression, and discusses how these drugs work, possible side effects, long-term effects, and how to deal with dependency or addiction to them.
Includes bibliographical references and index.
 ISBN 1-4034-0821-1
 1. Psychotropic drugs--Juvenile literature. 2. Analgesics--Juvenile literature. [1. Psychotropic drugs. 2. Analgesics. 3. Drugs.] I. Title. II. Series.
 RM315 .D885 2003
 615'.78--dc21
                         2002010941

Acknowledgments
The author and publisher are grateful to the following for permission to reproduce copyright material:
Cover photograph: Helen King/Corbis.
pp. 1, 38 BSIP, PIKO/Science Photo Library; pp. 4, 32 Damien Lovegrove/Science Photo Library; p. 7 Jose Luis Pelaz/Corbis; pp. 8, 9 Bettmann/Corbis; pp. 10–11 Adam Hart-Davis/Science Photo Library; pp. 13, 17 (top) David Hoffmann Photo Library; pp. 12, 25 Bob Daemmrich, Image Works/Topham; p. 15 Sally and Richard Greenhill; p. 17 (bottom), 30 Reuters/Popperfoto; pp. 18, 21, 35 Image Works/Topham; p. 23 Helen King/Corbis; p. 24 Stephen Welstead, LWA/Corbis; p. 27 Arlene Collins, Image Works/Topham; pp. 28, 40 CC Studio/Science Photo Library; p. 29 Nancy Richmond, Image Works/Topham; p. 36 Nils Jorgensen/Rex Features; p. 37 Arthur Trees/Science Photo Library; p. 39 Sierakowski, SEN/Rex Features; pp. 41, 43, 46 Oscar Burriel/Science Photo Library; p. 44 Isopress Senepart, SEN/Rex Features; p. 47 Robert Huntzinger/Corbis; p. 48 David Woods/Corbis; p. 49 SIPA/Rex Features; p. 51 Topham.

Every effort has been made to contact copyright holders of any material reproduced in this book. Any omissions will be rectified in subsequent printings if notice is given to the publishers.

Our special thanks to Pamela G. Richards, M.Ed., for her help in the preparation of the book.

Some words appear in bold, **like this.** You can find out what they mean by looking in the glossary.

Contents

Painkillers and Tranquilizers 4
What Are Painkillers and Tranquilizers? 6
The History of Painkillers 8
The History of Tranquilizers 10
What Is Pain? 12
How Do Painkillers Work? 14
Types of Painkillers 16
Side Effects of Painkillers 18
Why Do People Need Tranquilizers? 20
Types of Tranquilizers 24
Side Effects of Tranquilizers 26
Tranquilizers and Antidepressants 28
Tranquilizers as Street Drugs 30
When Drugs Can Be Avoided 32
Dependence 34
Stopping Tranquilizers 42
Alternatives to Drugs 46
Legal Matters 48
People Who Can Help 50
Information and Advice 52
More Books to Read 53
Glossary 54
Index 56

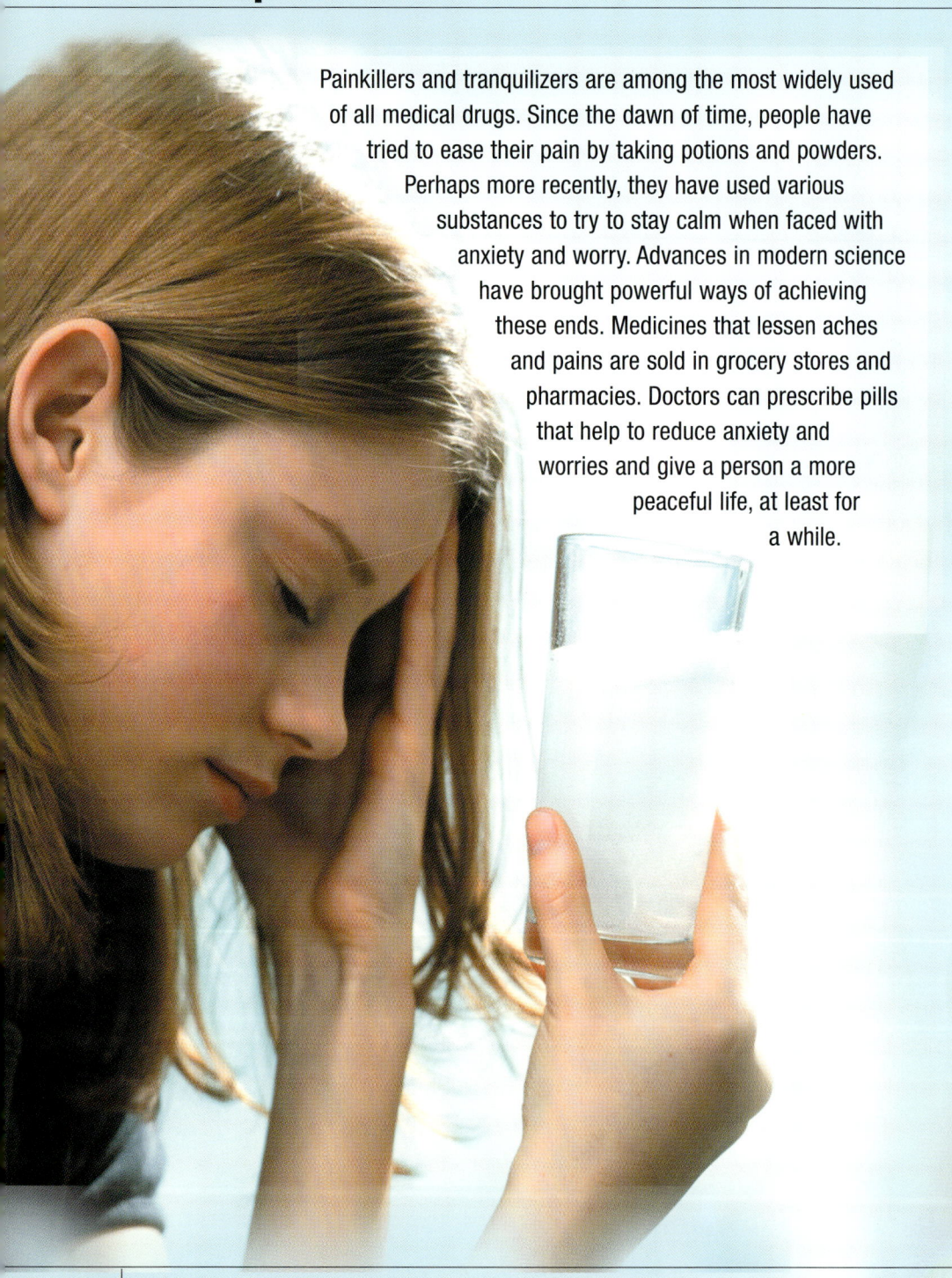

Painkillers and Tranquilizers

Painkillers and tranquilizers are among the most widely used of all medical drugs. Since the dawn of time, people have tried to ease their pain by taking potions and powders. Perhaps more recently, they have used various substances to try to stay calm when faced with anxiety and worry. Advances in modern science have brought powerful ways of achieving these ends. Medicines that lessen aches and pains are sold in grocery stores and pharmacies. Doctors can prescribe pills that help to reduce anxiety and worries and give a person a more peaceful life, at least for a while.

Obtaining the drugs

Some painkillers, usually the less powerful types, are available **over-the-counter (OTC)**. This means they can be obtained without a doctor's prescription, usually from a pharmacy or grocery store. Other painkillers, generally the stronger versions, are available only from a pharmacy, with a doctor's prescription. Tranquilizers are obtained mainly by prescription. However, both groups of drugs sometimes make their appearance on the street as part of the illegal drug trade.

Both painkillers and tranquilizers are available in a wide range of types and strengths. These are known by various names, including the chemical name of the drug, and the trade or brand name that is used by the drug manufacturer. The variety of names can be extremely confusing.

The dangers

Drugs such as painkillers and tranquilizers have brought many benefits to many people. But, like other medicinal substances, they can also cause unwanted effects and problems.

One problem is **overdose.** An overdose of any drug is harmful, but with some painkillers it can be deadly. Another problem is **dependence.** This is especially risky with certain tranquilizers. Also, painkillers and tranquilizers can interact with each other, or with other drugs such as alcohol, to threaten both physical and mental health. In rare cases, the result may be fatal.

As with any drug, people taking painkillers or tranquilizers should take great care. This applies both to prescribed and over-the-counter types. Sometimes a person may worry that any benefit of the drug will be outweighed by **side effects.** A pharmacist or doctor can give information about such matters. There may be a range of nondrug choices for dealing with the person's difficulties, such as a change of lifestyle, counseling, or a **complementary therapy.**

What Are Painkillers and Tranquilizers?

Painkillers or pain-relievers are also called **analgesics.** They help to reduce or ease pain, although they may not get rid of it entirely. Some types, like **aspirin** and **acetaminophen** (more commonly known as Tylenol), are available without a doctor's prescription. This is because they are well-established and relatively safe. They are used to treat common ailments such as backache, headache, and toothache. But, like any other drug, they can be dangerous if taken in the wrong dose. They may also cause **side effects** in certain people.

More powerful painkillers

Stronger painkillers can only be obtained with a doctor's prescription. Most contain **morphine** or morphine-like substances. Morphine is a natural substance obtained from certain kinds of poppy flowers. Most of these stronger morphine-type painkillers are known scientifically as **opiates** or **opioids.** (This group of drugs also includes **heroin** and **opium.**) Under supervision of a doctor, they may be used by someone recovering from an operation in a hospital, or by a person suffering from a serious, painful illness such as cancer or arthritis.

Morphine-based painkillers can be extremely dangerous. They have various side effects and the user risks **dependence.** So morphine-based painkillers are considered **controlled drugs**—they can only be prescribed and possessed with special permission.

Tranquilizers

Tranquilizers alter people's moods. They are usually prescribed by a doctor for a short period. These drugs are for people suffering from great anxiety, worry, nervousness, or sleeplessness. Most tranquilizers have a calming or **sedative** effect. They help people to feel less worried, upset, and agitated, and more positive and able to cope with life. Some types reduce extreme highs and lows of emotion.

In general, tranquilizers work quickly and last for a few hours, occasionally longer. Someone who feels particularly anxious or agitated could take a tranquilizer and start feeling the benefits almost immediately. This is why these drugs can help people get to sleep.

7

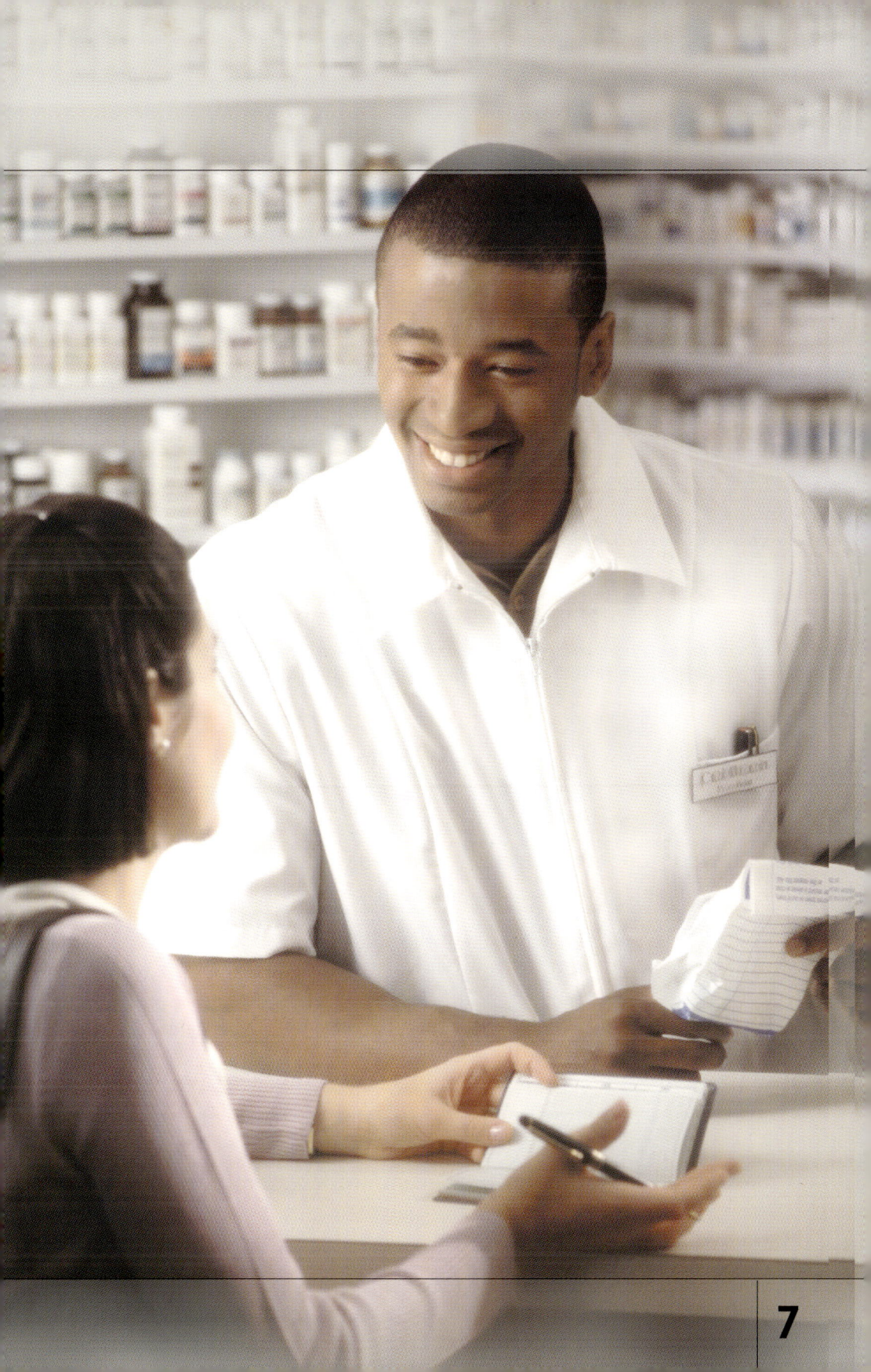

The History of Painkillers

Before modern scientific medicine, people used natural substances they found around them to treat illness and ease pain. Certain kinds of plant leaves, flowers, stems, and roots have been used through the ages for their medicinal qualities. Some of these natural medicines, if used incorrectly, were dangerous or even deadly. But others proved to be very effective, and many of the synthetic (artificial) drugs available today are based on them.

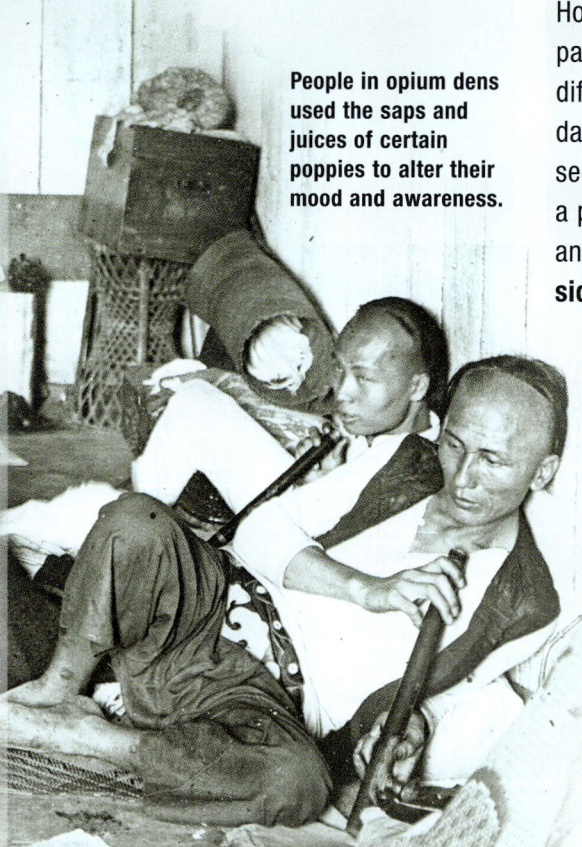

People in opium dens used the saps and juices of certain poppies to alter their mood and awareness.

The first painkillers

The first doctors were shamans or priests. They used rituals, such as chanting and dancing, along with natural medicines to treat the sick and relieve pain. The powerful natural painkiller **opium** has been used for thousands of years. Other medicinal plants that can have pain-reducing effects include ginseng, mandragora, hemlock, and willow bark.

However, these types of natural painkillers were often unreliable, difficult to use, and sometimes dangerous. In some cases they hardly seemed to work at all. In other cases, a person could accidentally be given an **overdose** and suffer severe **side effects** or even die.

In the 1800s, one of the most common painkillers was laudanum, which was made from opium and alcohol. Unfortunately, many people became **dependent** on it. Another traditional way to relieve pain, such as during an operation, was to give patients large amounts of alcohol. This helped to dull pain. In fact, it often did far more, and made the patient so drunk that he or she fell asleep and felt nothing.

Pain during operations

Pain relief during operations was more effective in the late 19th century. Doctors and dentists began to use gases, such as ether and chloroform, to put their patients to sleep during surgery. Today there are many kinds of **anesthetics** that reduce feeling and pain.

Aspirin was the first painkiller suitable for general use by people with common aches and pains. In 1899, it was marketed by the Swiss company Bayer as "the wonder drug that works wonders." In fact, aspirin is one of the oldest painkillers. The chemical that has the painkilling effect is known as salicylate. It is found in the bark of certain trees, such as willow. Its pain-relieving qualities have been known for 2,500 years.

> **Pain is inevitable; suffering is optional.**

(A traditional saying that means we all suffer pain, but the way we deal with it, and the amount of suffering it causes, are more individual matters.)

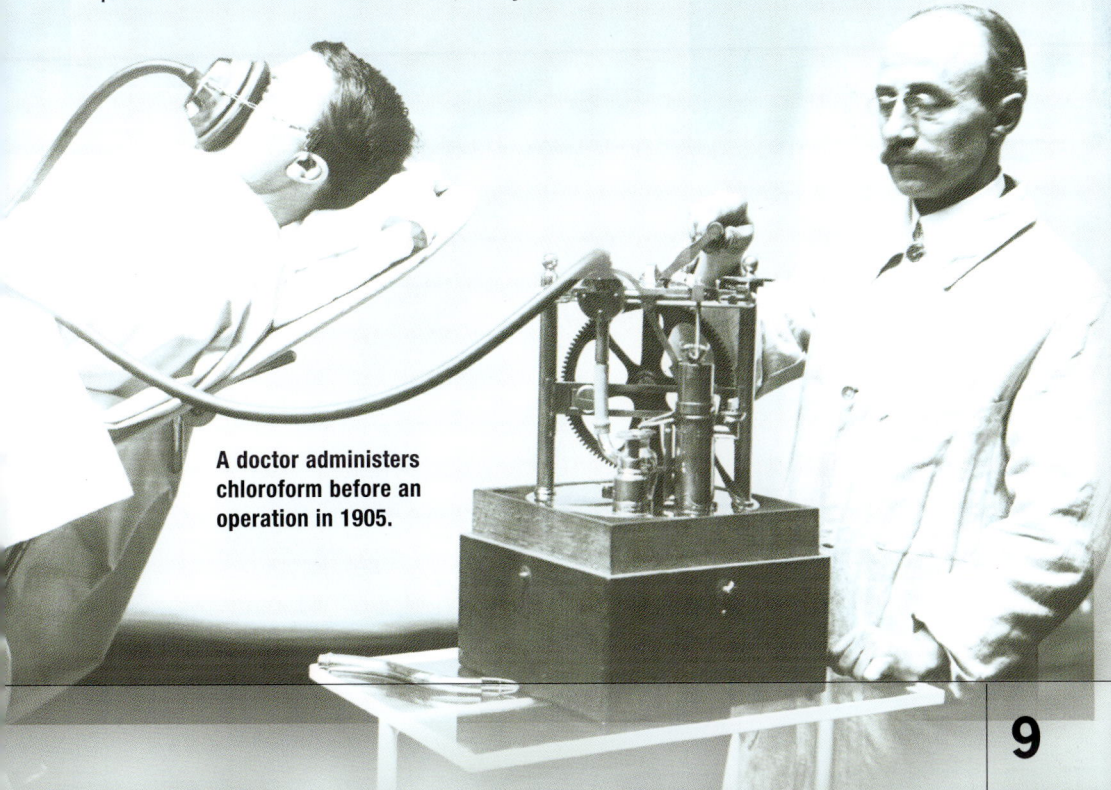

A doctor administers chloroform before an operation in 1905.

The History of Tranquilizers

For thousands of years people have used natural substances to alter their mood and make them feel more content. To some extent, alcohol can have this effect, acting to calm an agitated person. Substances were also extracted from coca leaves and **opium** poppies for their mind-altering qualities.

Many herbal plants have been used as natural remedies for anxiety and to help people sleep. They include valerian root and chamomile tea. These and others were used by people who "suffered from nerves" or who were "high-strung." Such natural medicines were also used by people who had **nervous breakdowns.** Many of these herbs are still used today.

The modern era

The first modern tranquilizer made by chemical methods was chlordiazepoxide. It was developed by chemist Leo Sternbach in 1957. Tests showed it had a **sedative** and calming effect. It was marketed in 1960 as **Librium,** and soon became one of the best-selling medicines in the world.

Chlordiazepoxide belongs to a group of tranquilizers called **benzodiazepines,** or benzos. Its discovery led to the development of other tranquilizers in the group. One is diazepam, stronger than Librium and marketed as **Valium.** Another is nitrazepam, with the trade name **Mogadon.**

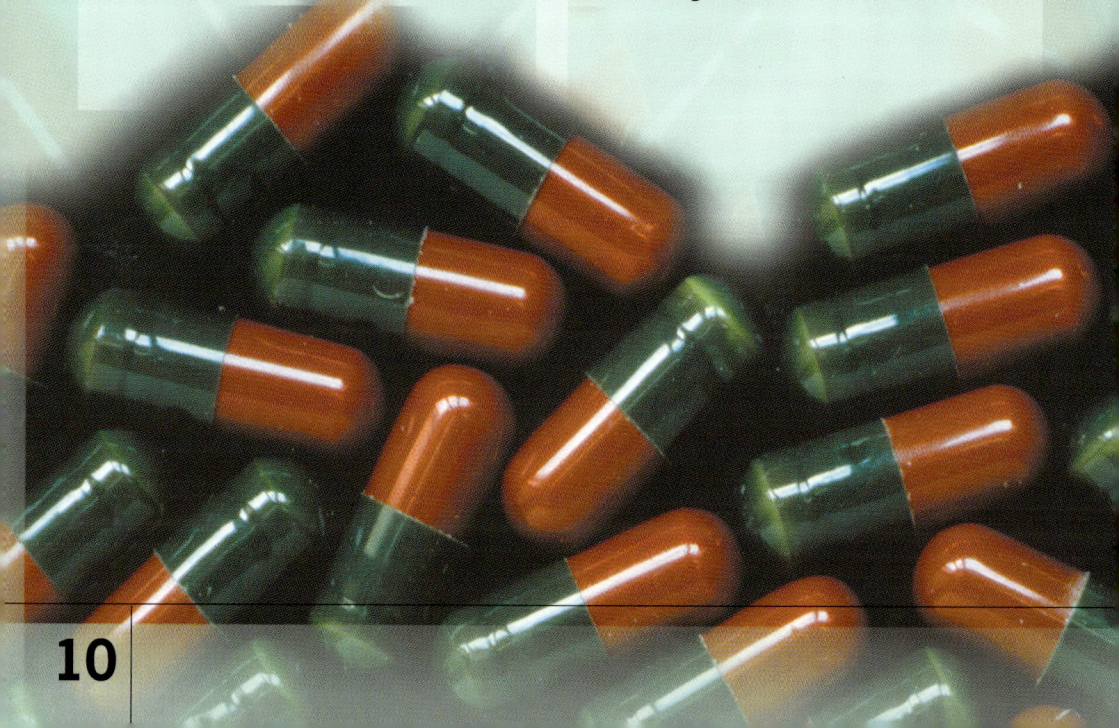

Happy pills

During the 1960s and 1970s, benzodiazepine tranquilizers were hailed as safe, effective pills for a wide range of problems, especially the stresses and strains of daily life. They gained nicknames such as "happy pills" and "mother's little helpers." This was because they were often prescribed for mothers with young children who had to cope with busy lives.

A drug company advertisement aimed at doctors showed such a mother pinned inside a prison of brooms and mops. The slogan was "You can't set her free, but you can help her feel less anxious." However, as the prescriptions for benzodiazepines increased, so did the problems they caused, especially **dependence**.

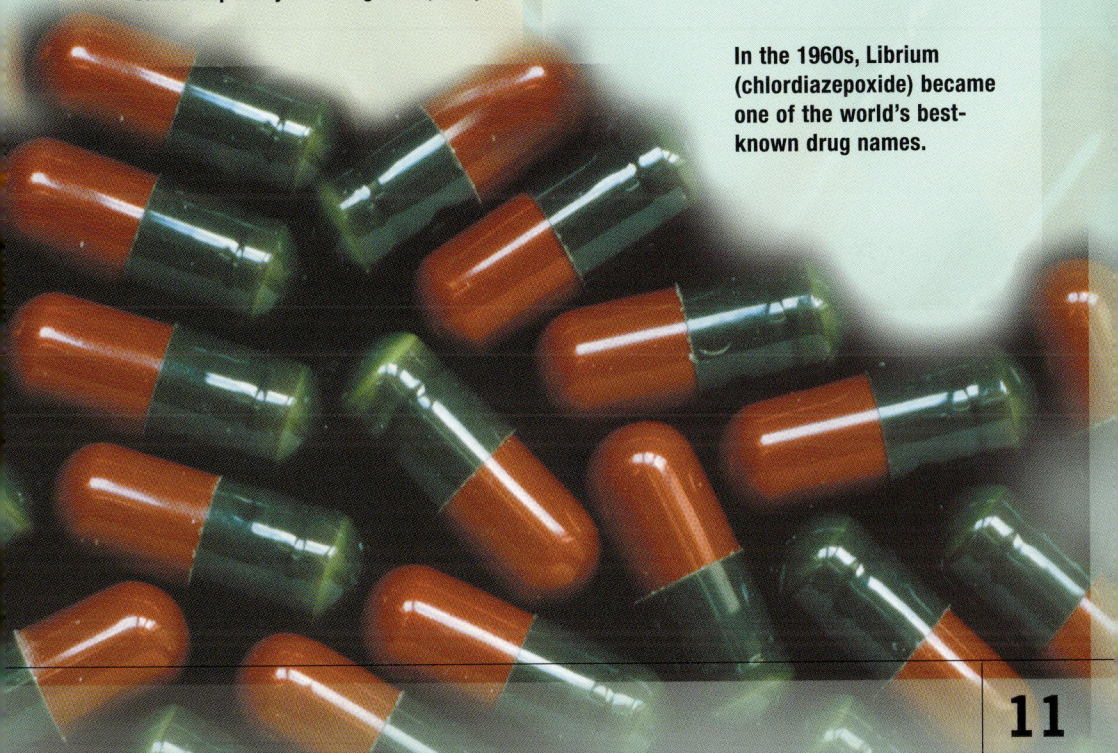

> "She goes running for the shelter,
> Of a mother's little helper,
> And it helps her on her way,
> Gets her through her busy day."
>
> (From "Mother's Little Helper," a song about benzodiazepines by The Rolling Stones, 1967)

In the 1960s, Librium (chlordiazepoxide) became one of the world's best-known drug names.

What Is Pain?

You are the only person who can feel your pain. This makes describing pain difficult. We use words such as sharp, hot, stabbing, shooting, or dull. But how do we know that we are all using these descriptions in the same way? Also, when does a slight ache, twinge, or discomfort become a real pain? If several people had exactly the same painful condition, would they all feel the same type and amount of pain? There is no scientific method of comparing the amount or severity of pain between different people.

Inside the body, pain exists as a series of tiny electrical signals called nerve impulses. These are made by tiny nerve endings known as pain sensors, usually when damage has been caused to a body part, such as after stubbing a toe. The signals travel along nerves to the brain. The person becomes aware of them in his or her mind as a painful sensation.

Types of pain

- A sharp, sudden pain, such as when you stub your toe, is sometimes called protective pain. It is a reaction to danger, like an early warning system.
- The throbbing, longer-lasting pain that sets in after a more serious injury is called reparative pain. It means damage is being repaired.
- Neuropathic pain is a severe, long-term pain as a result of damage to the nervous system itself.

The need for pain

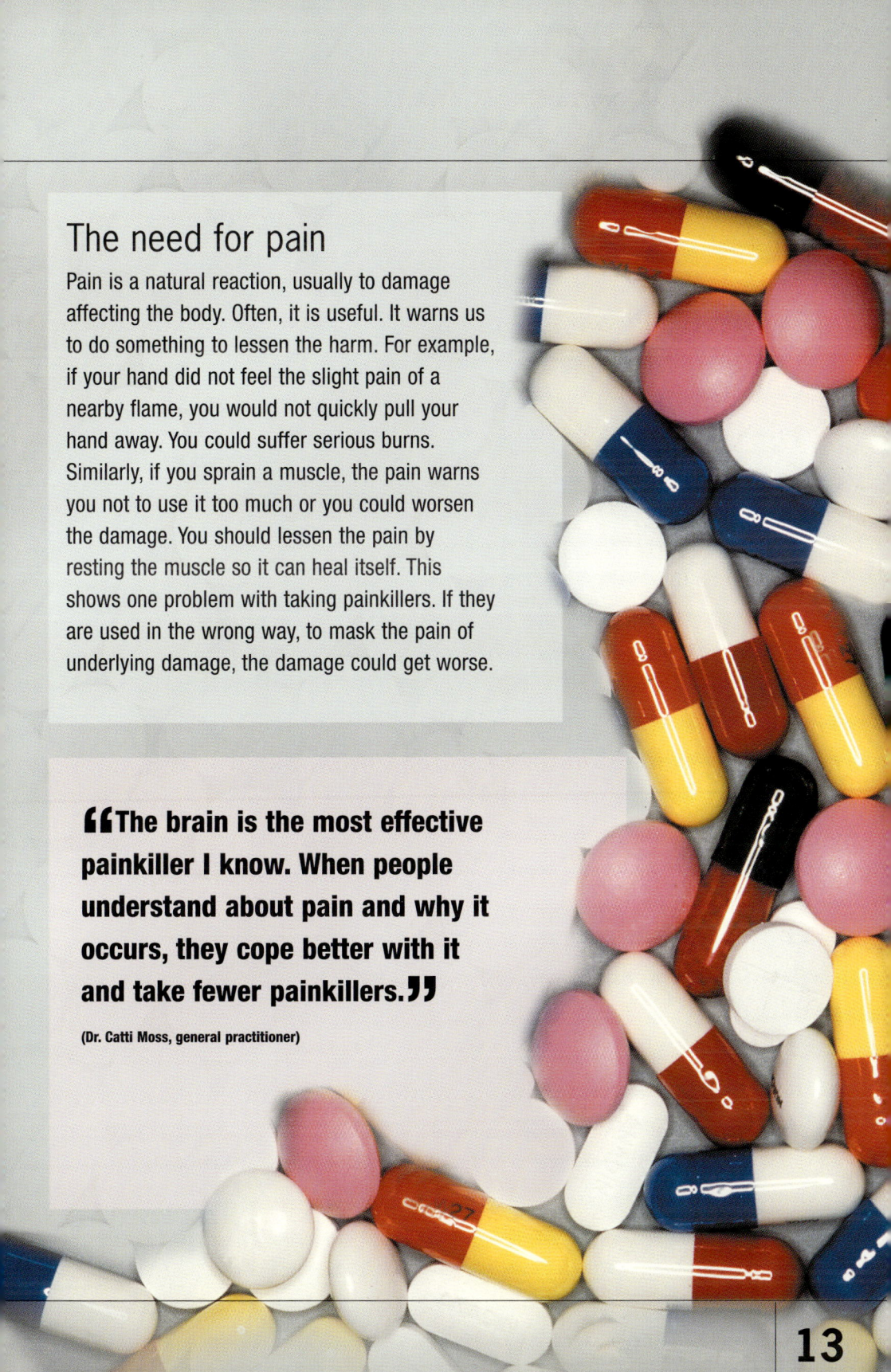

Pain is a natural reaction, usually to damage affecting the body. Often, it is useful. It warns us to do something to lessen the harm. For example, if your hand did not feel the slight pain of a nearby flame, you would not quickly pull your hand away. You could suffer serious burns. Similarly, if you sprain a muscle, the pain warns you not to use it too much or you could worsen the damage. You should lessen the pain by resting the muscle so it can heal itself. This shows one problem with taking painkillers. If they are used in the wrong way, to mask the pain of underlying damage, the damage could get worse.

"The brain is the most effective painkiller I know. When people understand about pain and why it occurs, they cope better with it and take fewer painkillers."

(Dr. Catti Moss, general practitioner)

How Do Painkillers Work?

Painkillers do not kill pain by removing the cause of it. If someone suffers a hard hit on the arm, then the area is painful. There might be swelling and a bruise. If that person takes a painkiller, the pain lessens. But the damage, swelling, and bruising are still there. The actual cause of the pain only fades away as the area heals and repairs itself.

Stopping pain signals

Most painkillers interfere with the way that the signals for pain pass along the body's nerves, or change how the brain deals with the signals.

Some types of painkillers affect the pain sensors that detect damage and produce the signals in the first place. Other painkillers dull the signals as they travel along nerves to the brain. In both cases, the full signals do not reach the brain itself.

The other main group of painkillers works on the brain itself. The nerve signals from a painful area reach the brain. But then they are altered or blocked. This affects the way the sensation of pain is recognized and felt in the mind.

Anti-inflammatories

Some painkillers, such as **aspirin,** relieve pain in other ways, too. They are **anti-inflammatory.** This means they reduce the swelling, redness, heat, and soreness of inflammation where the body is suffering damage. Other painkillers work differently than aspirin. These differences show the importance of matching the type of painkiller to the nature and cause of the pain.

Julie's story

Fourteen-year-old Julie suffered from severe menstrual (period) pain that lasted two or three days. After a talk with her family doctor, she tried changes in her diet and her lifestyle, including exercise. The problem lessened, but still caused discomfort. At the next visit, her doctor suggested a prescription painkiller. However, Julie did not want to be hooked on a strong prescription drug that she felt might cause long-term problems. So the doctor suggested further changes in lifestyle, especially in diet and coping with stress. The doctor said that Julie could try taking **ibuprofen** a day before her period was due, if necessary. Now Julie feels much less pain, and she does not need to visit her doctor regularly for a prescription.

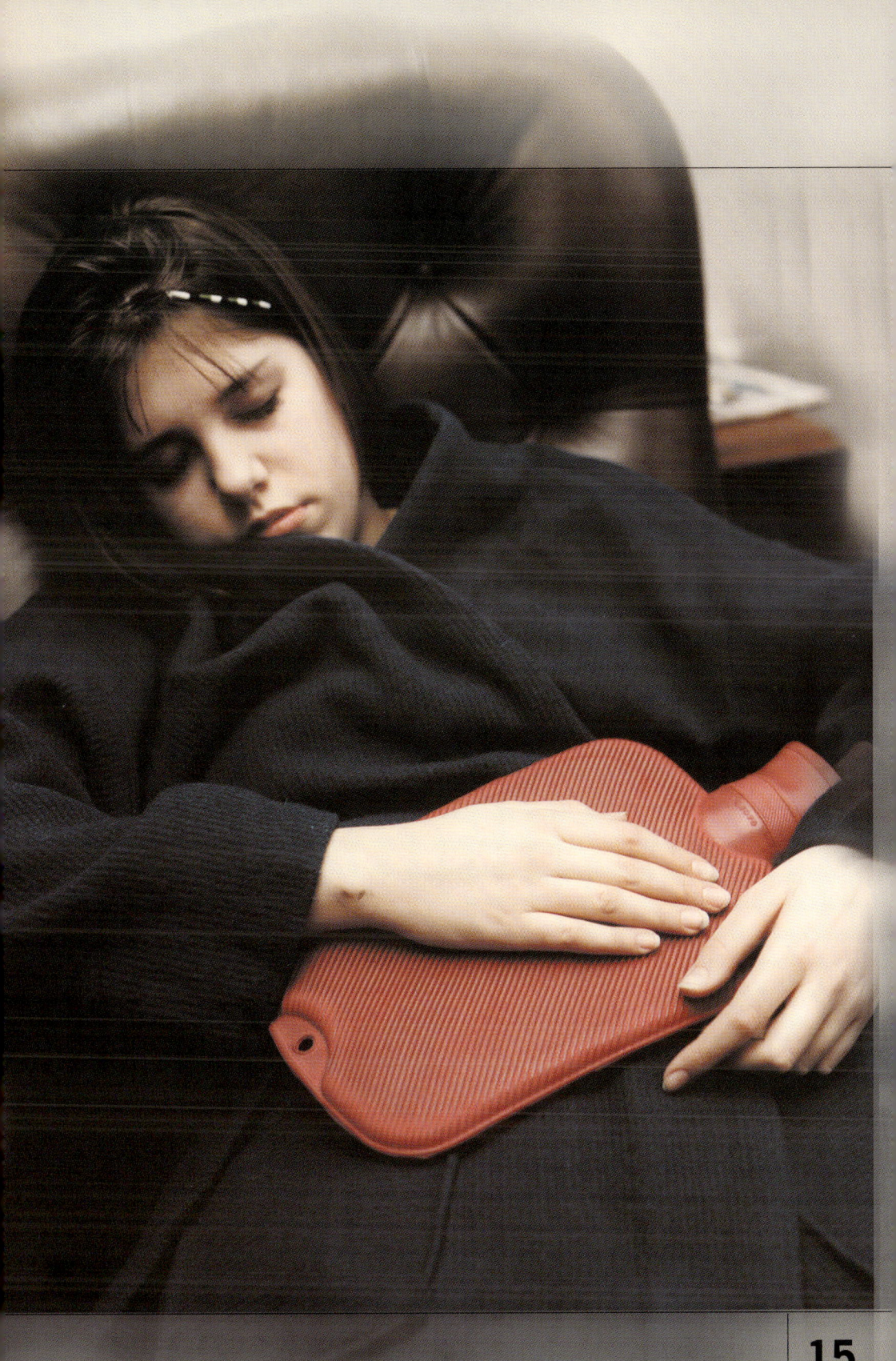

Types of Painkillers

Aspirin is a common painkiller. It reduces pain in several ways. One way is by stopping the production of natural body chemicals called prostaglandins. These are made in any body part that is injured or damaged. Normally, their job is to alert the brain that damage has occurred. They affect the pain sensors and send signals to the brain. If prostaglandins cannot be made, the messages are not sent and the person does not feel pain. Aspirin also helps to reduce inflammation in joints and muscles. The inflammation itself causes pain, so reducing it lessens the pain.

NSAIDs

Aspirin is known as a non-steroidal **anti-inflammatory** drug **(NSAID)**. **Ibuprofen** is another NSAID and works in a similar way. NSAIDs are often prescribed for painful, long-term conditions such as arthritis, neck pain, or backache, in which keeping down inflammation is also important. There is another large group of drugs known as steroids that also act against inflammation. But steroids are very different in chemical form to NSAIDs, and work in different ways.

Acetaminophen

The most common **over-the-counter** painkiller is **acetaminophen.** It relieves pain and, like aspirin, also reduces fever and brings down body temperature. Acetaminophen has few **side effects,** and is usually safe for both adults and children. But unlike NSAIDs such as aspirin, acetaminophen does not have anti-inflammatory effects. Also, it is extremely dangerous if an **overdose** is taken.

Powerful painkillers

The group of powerful painkillers called **opiate-opioids** includes **morphine, codeine,** methadone, and **heroin.** These drugs are sometimes called **narcotic analgesics** because they can bring on narcosis (sleep so deep that it becomes unconsciousness). Most carry serious risks, including **dependence.** Their use is therefore closely controlled, and doctors can only prescribe them in carefully monitored cases, such as for seriously ill hospital patients.

The business of growing poppies to produce drugs such as morphine and heroin still occurs, even though it is illegal in most places.

16

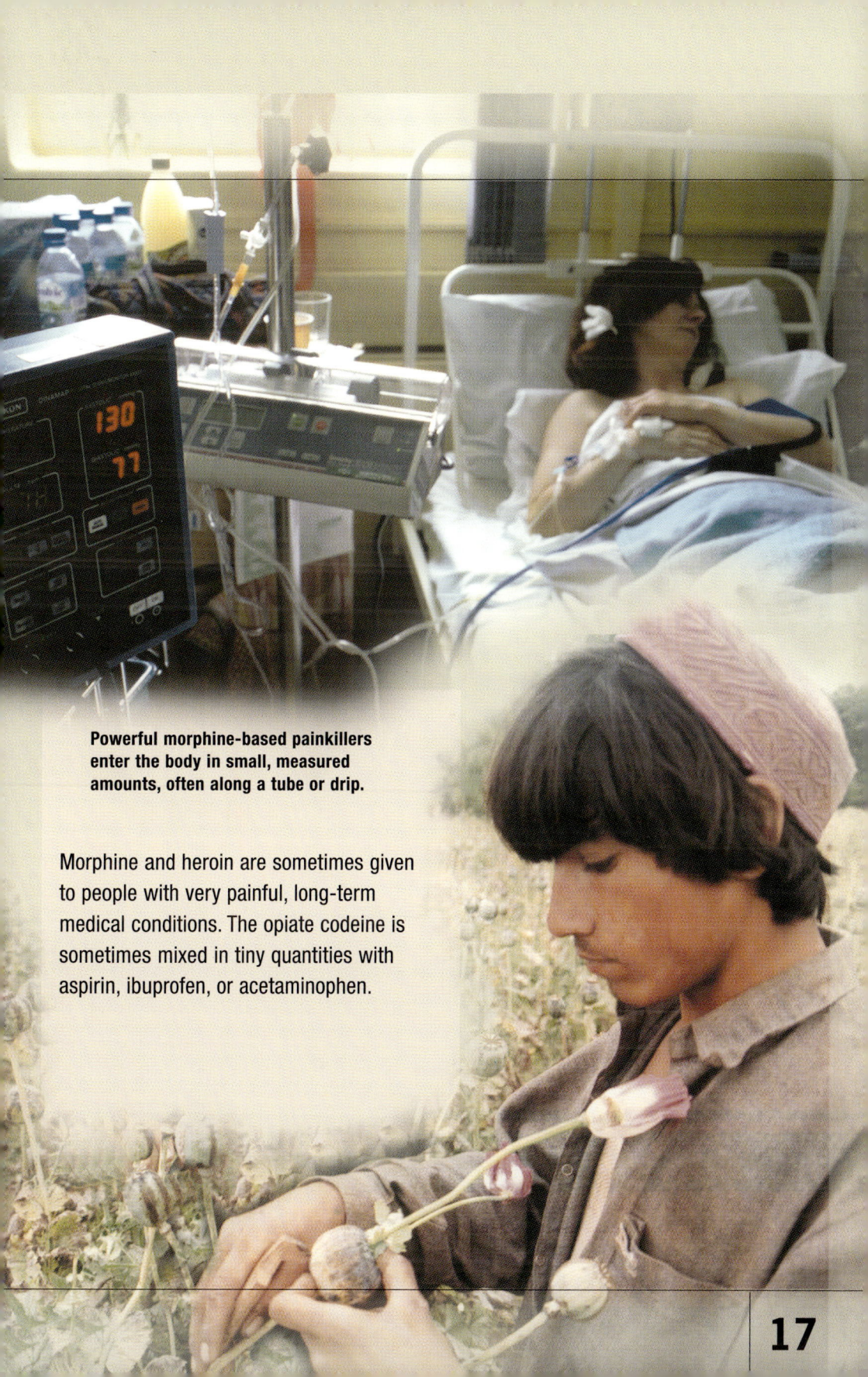

Powerful morphine-based painkillers enter the body in small, measured amounts, often along a tube or drip.

Morphine and heroin are sometimes given to people with very painful, long-term medical conditions. The opiate codeine is sometimes mixed in tiny quantities with aspirin, ibuprofen, or acetaminophen.

Side Effects of Painkillers

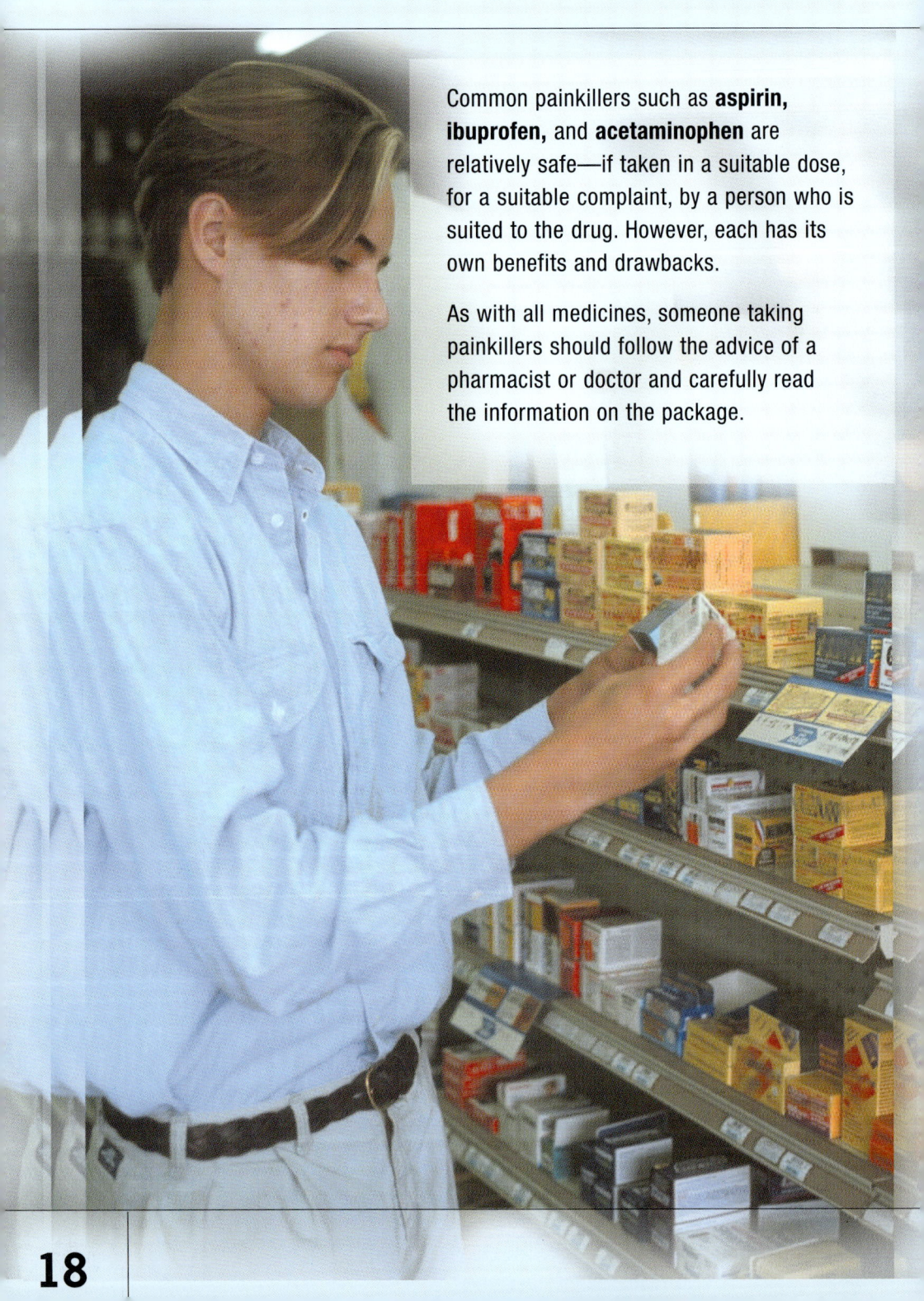

Common painkillers such as **aspirin, ibuprofen,** and **acetaminophen** are relatively safe—if taken in a suitable dose, for a suitable complaint, by a person who is suited to the drug. However, each has its own benefits and drawbacks.

As with all medicines, someone taking painkillers should follow the advice of a pharmacist or doctor and carefully read the information on the package.

Most drugs have **side effects.** This is especially true of drugs that alter the workings of the brain and nervous system. So, while the drug seems to solve one problem, it can be creating another. Some pills also react dangerously with other medicines and even with common foods and drinks.

Stomach bleeding

The most serious side effect of **over-the-counter NSAID** painkillers such as aspirin and ibuprofen is the risk of stomach bleeding. The drug attaches itself to important chemicals in the stomach, called enzymes, and prevents them from working. Every year a number of people become ill, and a few may die, after taking NSAID painkillers. Statistics in the United States show that the side effects of aspirin and other NSAIDs result in an estimated 16,000 deaths per year, mainly due to bleeding in the stomach. The risk is small, but significant. Such NSAIDs are not recommended for people who have suffered stomach ulcers or similar stomach problems in the past.

Dangers of aspirin

Aspirin should not be taken by people at risk of kidney or liver problems. Also, it is dangerous when mixed with alcohol. There have been claims that taking aspirin or ibuprofen can make it more likely for a pregnant woman to have a miscarriage (lose her baby). Usually the painkiller acetaminophen is more suitable for a woman expecting a baby.

Aspirin is not recommended for children under twelve years old. Acetaminophen can be used by children in small doses, and, in general, it has fewer side effects than NSAIDs. But acetaminophen has its own drawbacks. A major problem is the danger of an **overdose,** accidental or deliberate. It is possible to take a fatal overdose of any painkiller, but acetaminophen is especially risky because it can damage the liver very quickly. Unless immediate action is taken (within six to eight hours), this damage cannot be reversed. It may well lead to a slow and painful death.

Why Do People Need Tranquilizers?

Everybody feels anxious, agitated, worried, or upset at some time. People have problems such as passing exams, getting along with their family, finding a job, making friends, or losing a friend or close relative. Most of the time, we recover from these feelings naturally. After a while, new events and situations come along, and life looks more positive and fulfilling again.

Constant worry

For some people, worry and nervousness do not always have a particular cause. They have anxious feelings most of the time, often for no specific reason. They feel scared and jumpy and lack confidence. Even if things are going well, they worry that things will go wrong. They may expect the worst all the time.

For a few people, these feelings of anxiety, agitation, and worry become so powerful, and last so long, that they take over daily life. The person can no longer live a normal life. The anxiety affects sleeping and eating, home and work, and relationships with family and friends. It may begin to affect the person's health, too, so that he or she begins to suffer from infections and illnesses.

Drug treatment

If this stage is reached, a doctor may prescribe tranquilizers. The aim of the antianxiety drug treatment is to provide some breathing space. It enables the person to lose the agitation, worry, and nervousness and get back to calm, confident, and positive thoughts. It is like a push-start in the right direction. Gradually, the person can return to a more normal lifestyle. Hopefully, the drug will be needed for only a short time and the patient can stop taking it after a few weeks.

> **We have doctors, nurses, teachers, judges, and TV personalities among our clients. If you tried to sell them marijuana on a street corner, they'd be horrified. But many of them have stressful jobs, and these drugs make them feel calmer.**
>
> (David Greive, founder of Over-Count, an organization that helps people beat dependence on OTC drugs, 2000)

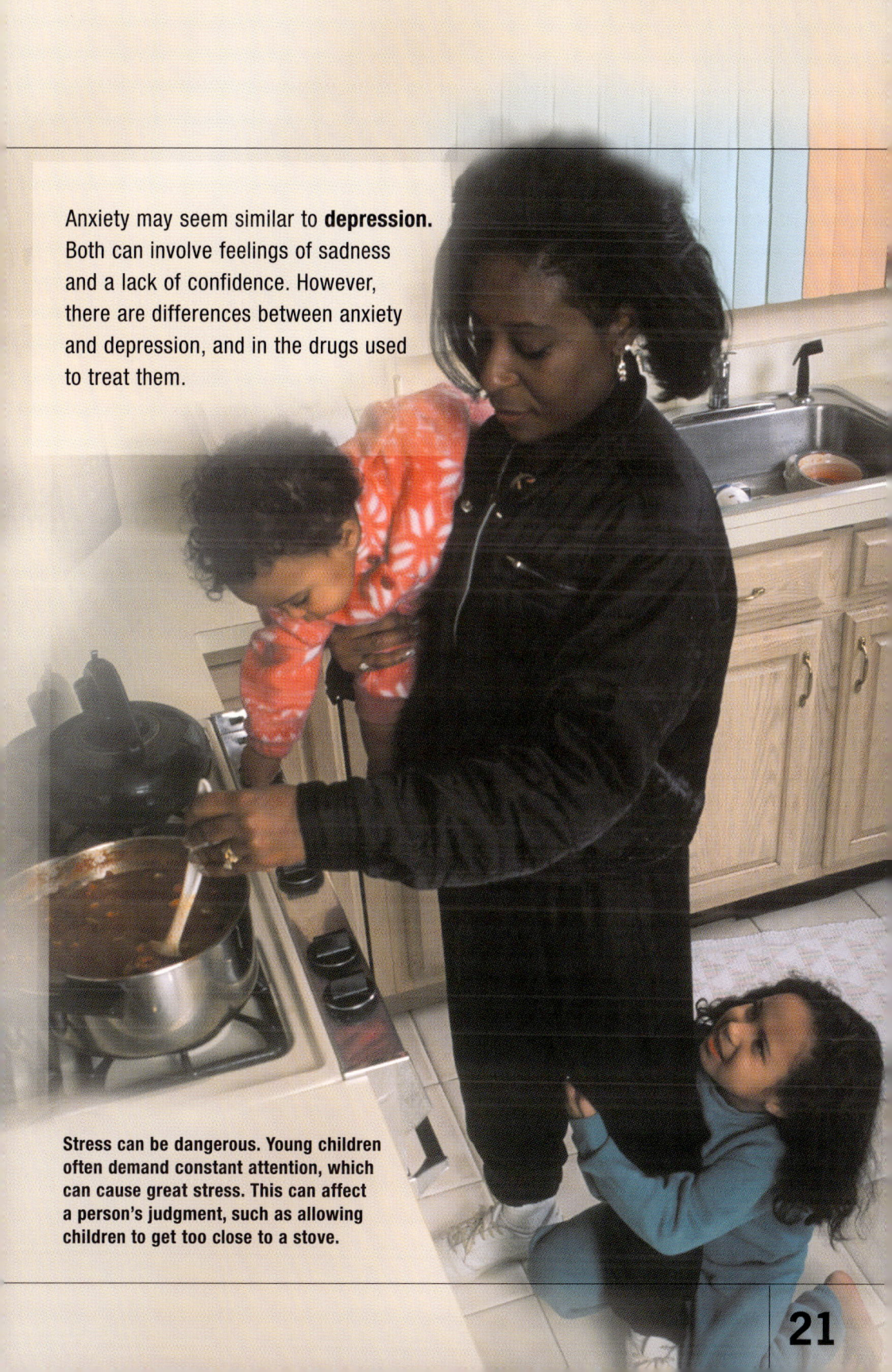

Anxiety may seem similar to **depression.** Both can involve feelings of sadness and a lack of confidence. However, there are differences between anxiety and depression, and in the drugs used to treat them.

Stress can be dangerous. Young children often demand constant attention, which can cause great stress. This can affect a person's judgment, such as allowing children to get too close to a stove.

Tranquilizers can be prescribed to almost anyone—salesclerks, professors, teachers, astronauts, and bricklayers. But a doctor would have to feel that the patient's anxiety and worry are severe, disabling, and distressing. It would be very unusual for a doctor to suggest tranquilizers before trying other courses of action.

For example, a tranquilizer would not help a young person at school who was nervous about an upcoming exam. It could seriously affect memory and ability to concentrate, and bring on feelings of being less alert and more tired. Often, with this type of worry, a talk with a teacher, counselor, or trusted advisor can help. An older person may worry about being forced to retire early. Again, there are other courses of action, including advice and training in new skills.

Women and men

Medical research shows that women are three times more likely than men to be prescribed tranquilizers. Nobody is quite sure why. One theory is that doctors are simply more likely to suggest tranquilizers to women rather than to men. Another theory is that men cope with stress and worry by bottling it up inside or pretending it is not important, so they are less likely to visit a doctor with this problem. Women are more likely to visit a doctor because they realize something is wrong and want to get it out into the open and deal with it as soon as possible.

However, research into **dependency** problems caused by tranquilizers can show a different picture. In one study, three times more men than women were dependent on tranquilizers. Many of the men did not obtain their tranquilizers by prescription, but from the illegal drug trade. They tended to use both tranquilizers and alcohol as a form

> **"Whatever the diagnosis—Librium."**
>
> (Drug company advertisement from the 1970s)

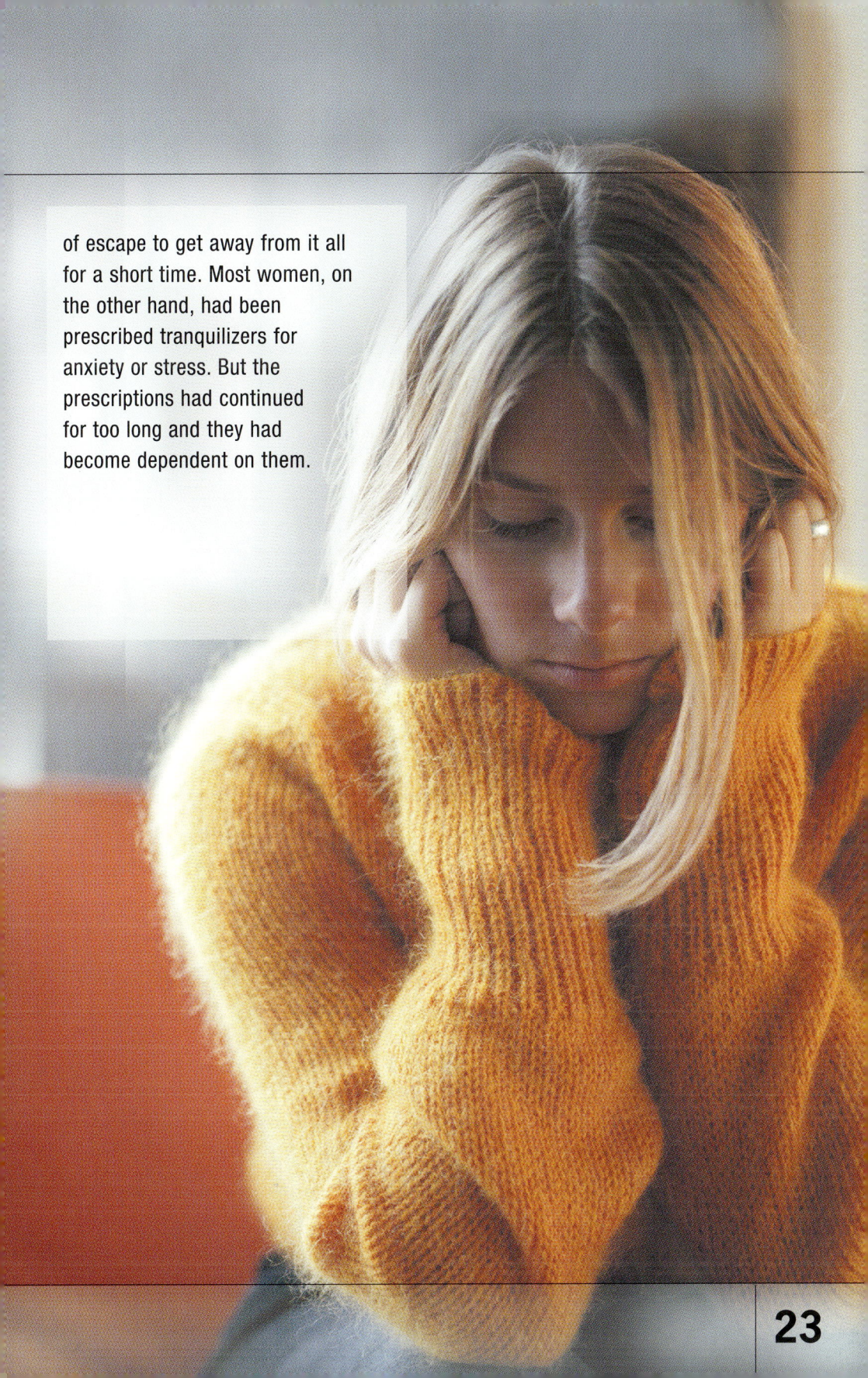

of escape to get away from it all for a short time. Most women, on the other hand, had been prescribed tranquilizers for anxiety or stress. But the prescriptions had continued for too long and they had become dependent on them.

Types of Tranquilizers

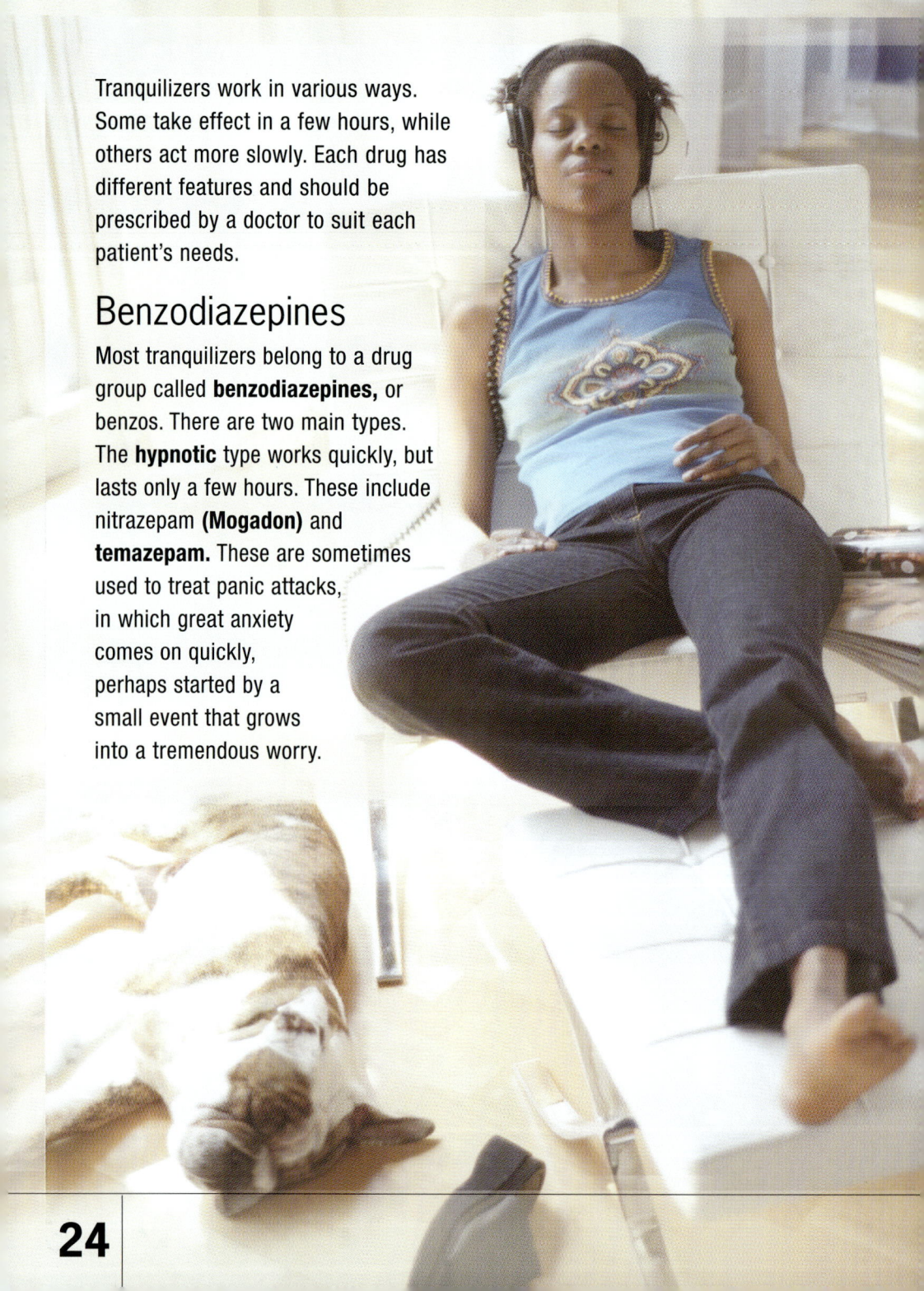

Tranquilizers work in various ways. Some take effect in a few hours, while others act more slowly. Each drug has different features and should be prescribed by a doctor to suit each patient's needs.

Benzodiazepines

Most tranquilizers belong to a drug group called **benzodiazepines,** or benzos. There are two main types. The **hypnotic** type works quickly, but lasts only a few hours. These include nitrazepam **(Mogadon)** and **temazepam.** These are sometimes used to treat panic attacks, in which great anxiety comes on quickly, perhaps started by a small event that grows into a tremendous worry.

The **anxiolytic** types include diazepam **(Valium)** and chlordiazepoxide **(Librium)**. Their effects take longer, but last longer, too.

Benzodiazepines are sometimes called minor tranquilizers. They produce feelings of calm and relaxation. Most also tend to make people feel sleepy, and they may be prescribed as sleeping pills.

Benzodiazepines tend to act on the parts of the brain involved with anxiety, but rarely on other parts. They should not alter a person's general behavior. However, some do affect other parts of the brain, and so have other uses, such as to control epilepsy.

Barbiturates

Barbiturates are powerful tranquilizer drugs rarely used today. **Dependence** on barbiturates occurs easily, and giving them up causes serious **withdrawal symptoms**. Also, the danger of a fatal **overdose** is high.

Barbiturates cause serious **tolerance** and dependence problems, comparable with those of hard drugs such as **heroin**. These problems are rare because barbiturates are strictly regulated. They are used medically only in rare cases. Also, as drugs of abuse, they have largely been replaced by other substances that users say are more powerful and have fewer immediate **side effects**.

Sean's story

Sean, aged sixteen, complained to his doctor that he could not sleep and always felt agitated and worried. His doctor suggested the feelings would pass and discussed positive new interests with Sean and his parents. But Sean's anxiety did not go away. So the doctor, with reluctance, prescribed seven pills of a mild tranquilizer. Sean could take one if he felt particularly bad.

At the same time, the doctor arranged for Sean to see a psychologist (an expert on the mind and behavior), who discovered the real reasons for Sean's anxiety. Sean was being bullied at school and had recently broken up with his girlfriend. After these reasons were revealed, Sean realized he did not need the pills. He managed to transfer to another school and gradually made new friends.

Side Effects of Tranquilizers

A common **side effect** of tranquilizers is a feeling of flatness or slowness. A person may feel the anxiety and worry lessen. But he or she may now be thinking more slowly, be less alert and aware, and be more confused and drowsy. These are known as **sedative** effects.

Tranquilizers have been blamed for affecting people's memory and ability to concentrate or make quick decisions, even though the people feel more confident and able to make good decisions. Tranquilizers can also lead to clumsiness and shakiness. The effects of some of the longer-lasting drugs continue into the following day.

Because of these various sedative effects, people who need to be wide awake and alert—such as pilots, truck drivers, and workers using complicated machinery—should not take tranquilizers. Indeed, their working conditions ban them from doing so.

Sleepwalking

When people use **benzodiazepines** for a long time, they may experience increasing feelings of tiredness and have less energy. Some people have called this "sleepwalking through life."

Many drugs can affect alertness and skilled coordination, and should be avoided when operating machinery.

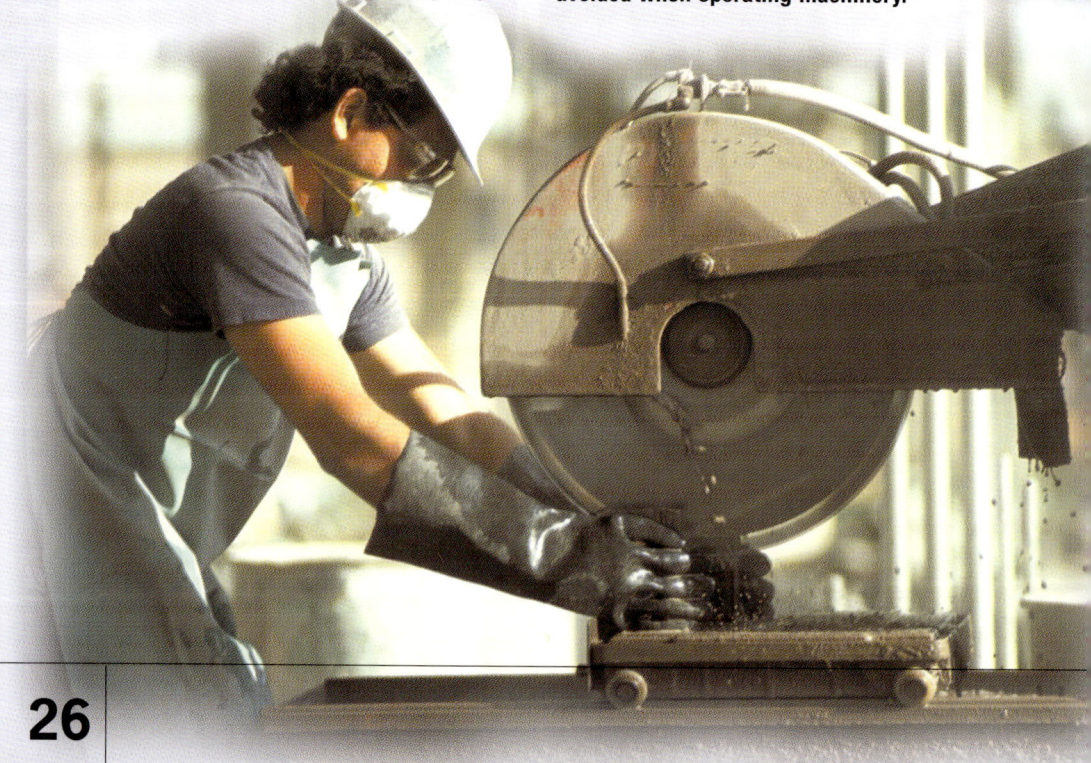

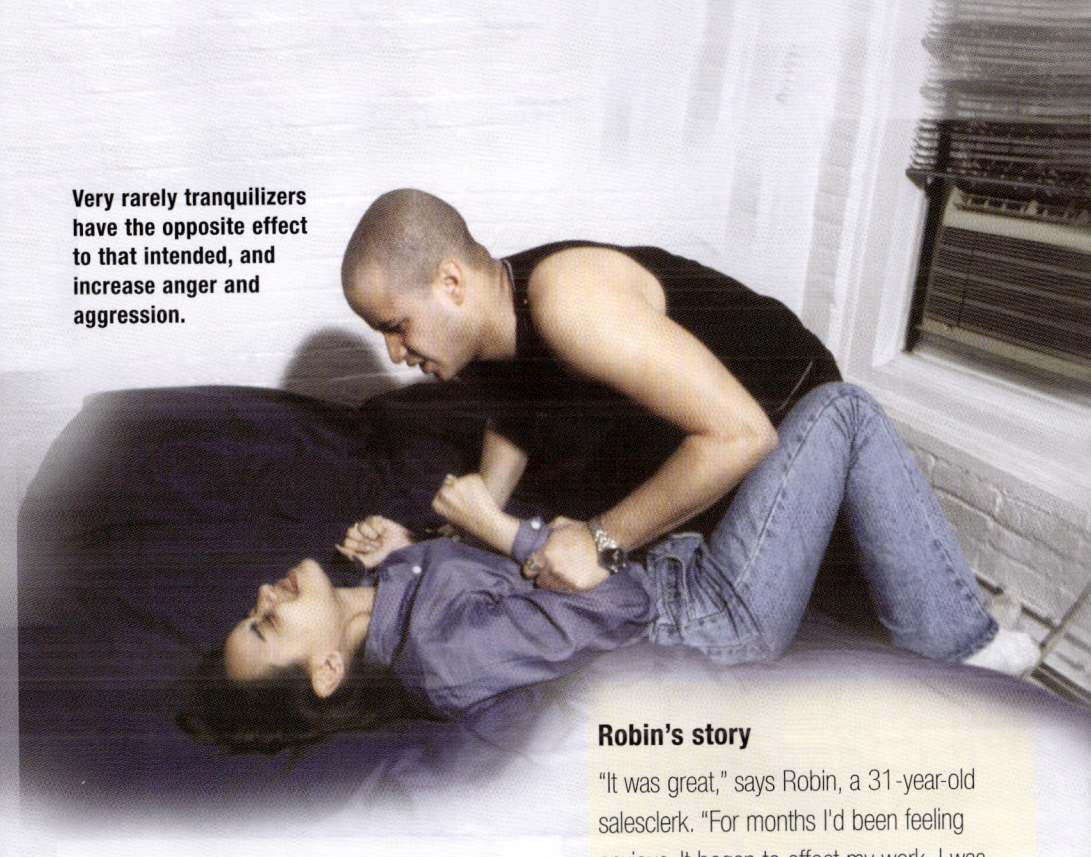

Very rarely tranquilizers have the opposite effect to that intended, and increase anger and aggression.

Also, many benzodiazepine users find that they are less anxious but, as a side effect, they begin to feel more **depressed.** If they are prescribed **antidepressants** as well, the antidepressants themselves can have side effects. It rapidly becomes difficult to sort out the real problems and symptoms from the side effects of the various drugs.

In a small number of cases, tranquilizers can have the opposite effect to what is intended. They make people more restless, angry, and aggressive. There is no way to predict if this will happen.

Robin's story

"It was great," says Robin, a 31-year-old salesclerk. "For months I'd been feeling anxious. It began to affect my work. I was warned about my attitude and making too many mistakes. That made the problem worse and life at home became very tense. Finally, I went to the doctor, and she prescribed a short course of tranquilizers. They worked, and the benefits began to affect my whole life. I could concentrate better. I spent more time dealing with what was happening, rather than worrying about what might happen. But I did feel myself slowing down and getting tired easily."

After four weeks, the doctor advised Robin to stop taking the drug. Robin was concerned, but he managed to get over the event. He is now much happier, less nervous, and more positive.

Tranquilizers and Antidepressants

Many people think of tranquilizers and **antidepressants** as almost the same thing. They are pills that help keep a person calm, happy, and relaxed. But they are very different types of drugs that work in different ways. Each type has its positive points and negative points.

Tranquilizers

As a summary, for comparison, tranquilizers are generally used to treat the symptoms of anxiety—feeling agitated, nervous, and restless. They act relatively quickly to make people calmer, less nervous, and more relaxed. Most tranquilizers work within a few hours and the effects wear off after a day or so. This means a person can take a tranquilizer now and then, as needed, to feel better when anxiety threatens. If feelings of anxiety fade, there may be no need to take a pill for weeks. But tranquilizers are **sedatives.** They can make people feel drowsy and confused. If they are taken regularly, day after day, they can make life seem drab, colorless, and boring.

In severe anxiety or during a panic attack, a person is extremely anxious. A casual thought or even a dream might trigger a whole series of worries about what might happen.

Antidepressants

Tranquilizers can be dangerously addictive. Antidepressants are less so. In recent years, more doctors have prescribed antidepressants, rather than tranquilizers, for anxiety. Some modern antidepressants are gradually replacing older tranquilizers. Indeed, the distinction between the conditions of **depression** and anxiety is also becoming more and more blurred.

Antidepressants, as their name suggests, treat depression. This usually involves feelings of great sadness, despair, and perhaps loneliness when all seems lost. There is often a lack of energy and little desire or motivation to be active and doing things. Antidepressant drugs do not cure depression, but they can take away the symptoms.

In contrast to tranquilizers, most types of antidepressants do not take effect quickly. In fact, many take roughly three to four weeks to start working. When they are stopped, it takes a long time for their effects to fade away.

Modern antidepressants do not make people feel drowsy or sedated as some tranquilizers do. But the antidepressant does not give a high or a lift either, with greatly raised mood and happiness. In fact, some people taking antidepressants notice hardly anything at all, except that they may feel less depressed.

29

Tranquilizers as Street Drugs

Many people experiment with street drugs. Some people try them once or a few times, but then stop using them. Others continue to take them for social reasons, perhaps with groups of friends or at a party or a bar. These people are often called **recreational users.** In a few cases, people continue to use a drug and become **dependent** on it.

Heroin and its dangers

Among the powerful painkillers called **opioids, heroin** can block out physical pain and also relieve emotional distress. It is usually made in small-scale illegal laboratories, rather than being stolen or otherwise obtained from medical sources. It can be mixed with all kinds of substances, such as chalk, talcum powder, or other drugs. Heroin tends to be smoked by new or younger experimental users, and injected by older, more experienced users. Its well-publicized dangers include dependence and the risk of serious infections such as HIV from used needles.

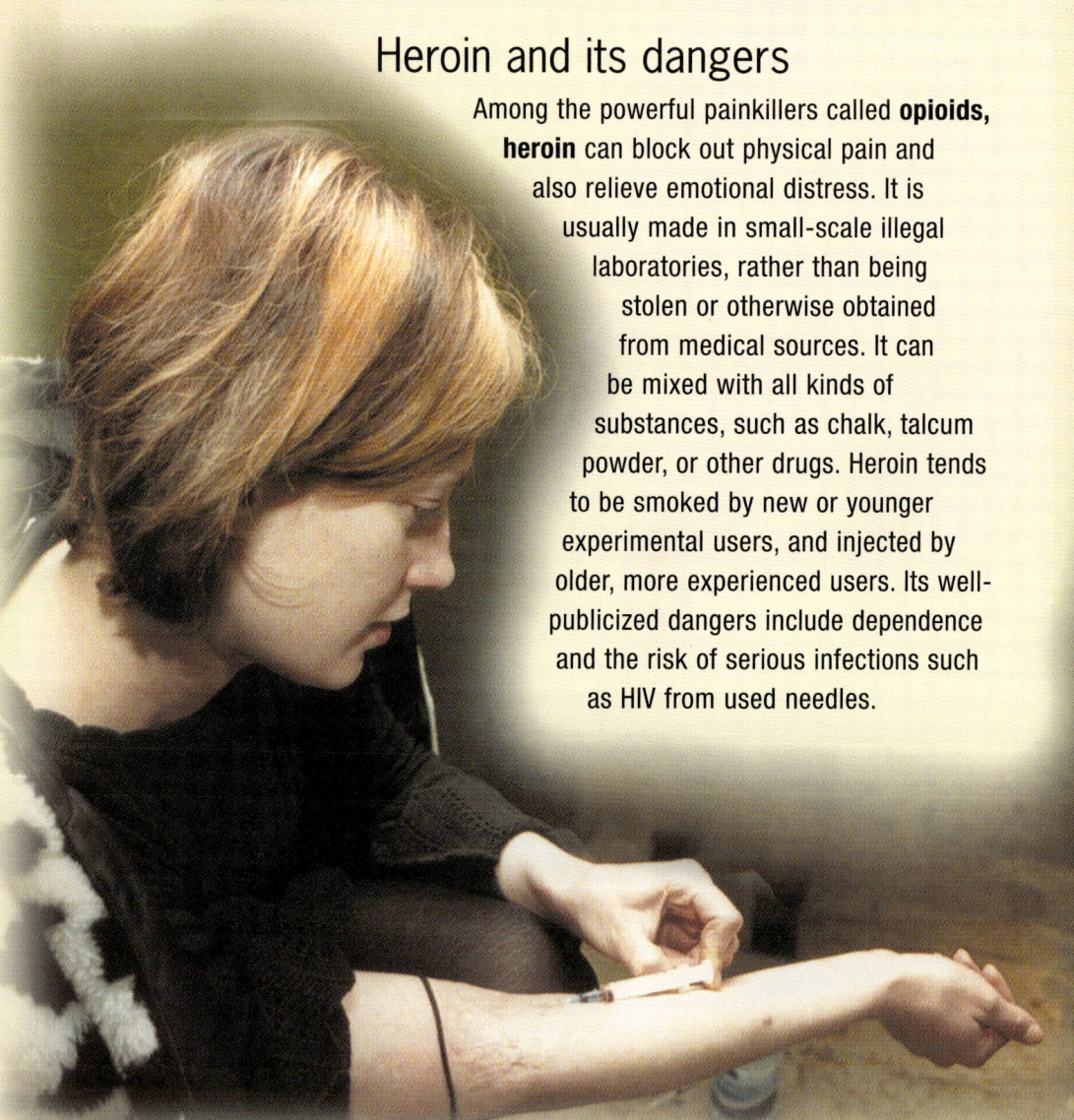

Misusing tranquilizers

Benzodiazepine tranquilizers became more common as street drugs in the 1980s. In some regions this partly resulted from shortages of heroin, as the police and other officials had increased success in seizing batches of the drug. **Temazepam** was one of the first most misused benzodiazepines, then diazepam **(Valium)** took its place. In 2001, an estimated three percent of the U.S. population used tranquilizers or pain relievers illegally.

Often these drugs are not taken alone, but with alcohol or opioids such as heroin, for a greater effect.

These combinations of drugs have led to an increase in substance abuse problems, because all three have a high risk of dependence. Drug-related deaths due to a combination of tranquilizer and alcohol abuse have also risen in recent years.

On the street

On the street, medicinal drugs often have different names:
- Tranquilizers are known as benzos or tranx.
- Nitrazepam (**Mogadon**) pills are moggies.
- Temazepam pills are green eggs, eggs, jellies, or tems.

Rohypnol—the date rape drug

The specialized tranquilizer flunitrazepam (Rohypnol) is known as the date rape drug. Slipped unnoticed into a drink, it can cause sleepiness, blackouts, and even short-term memory loss. The affected person is then at risk for rape or other abuse. There are severe penalties for illegally using or possessing this type of tranquilizer.

This young heroin user in Russia risks infection and drug dependence. When used as street drugs, benzodiazepines have similar risks.

When Drugs Can Be Avoided

It is difficult to control or track the use of painkillers because the common types are so widely available as **over-the-counter** medicines. Undoubtedly, many people take painkillers and tranquilizers when they do not really need them. For example, even if the underlying reason for a person's pain has been cured, she or he may not want to stop taking the drug in case the pain comes back. A few people even use painkillers to prevent pain in case of future accidents, saying "I might fall over and get hurt." Such unnecessary drug use puts the body at needless risk of any **side effects.**

Therapies

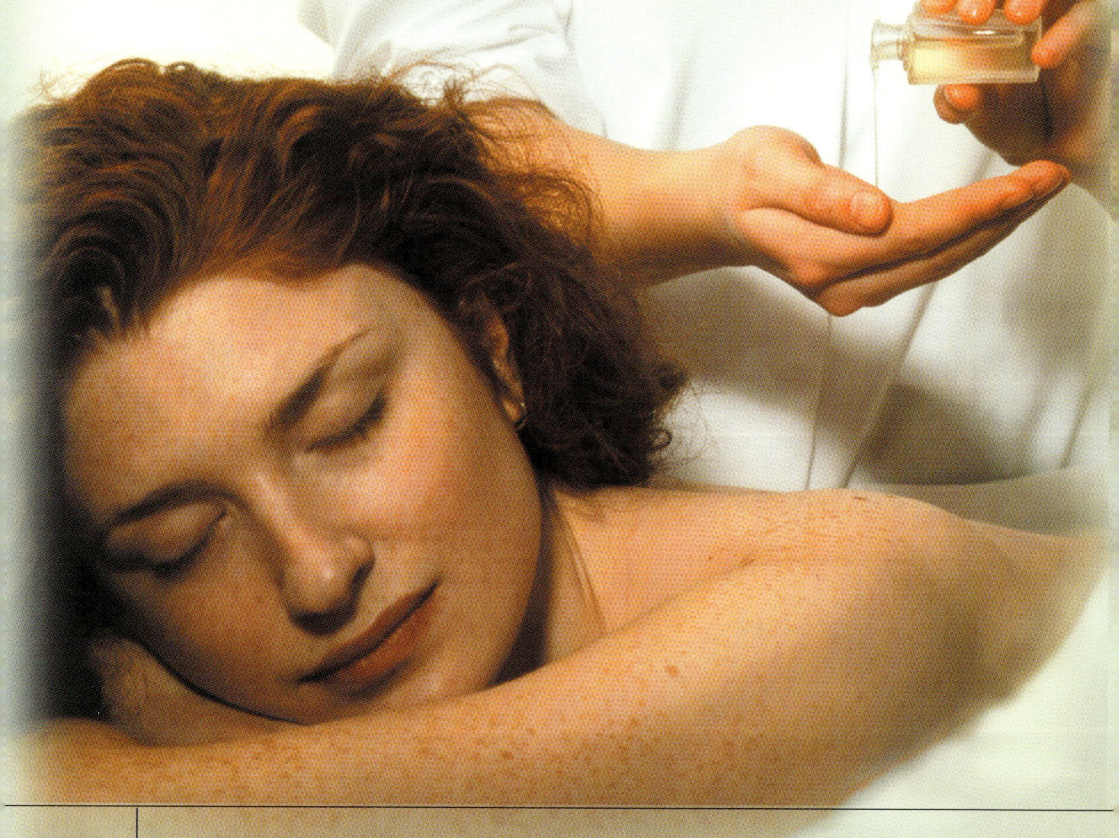

Tranquilizers are usually obtained under a doctor's prescription. But first, the doctor will normally try to find the underlying reason for the anxiety. He or she may then be able to suggest alternatives for treatment, rather than prescribing pills for the anxiety itself. A patient could visit a counselor or therapist, consider a change of lifestyle, or try a **complementary** treatment such as relaxation therapy or **hypnotherapy.** Therapies such as **psychotherapy,** in which problems are sorted out by talking about them, are also available.

A short-term solution

However, in some cases, a short course of tranquilizers may be appropriate, usually as a last resort.

Medical guidelines state that **benzodiazepines** should be prescribed only for severe and disabling anxiety or insomnia (sleeplessness) that is causing unacceptable stress. These tranquilizers should not be used for mild anxiety. They should be prescribed only in small amounts, enough for two to four weeks.

Patients can help themselves by asking their doctor about the lowest dose that may be effective, and the shortest time for which the drug can be taken. Also, when a prescription of tranquilizers is finished, patients can help themselves again. Is another prescription really needed? Can other changes be made to avoid the need for more drugs? If a patient feels there is no option but more tranquilizers, she or he is advised to see their doctor again for another discussion, rather than simply to ask for another prescription.

Many nondrug methods, such as getting a massage with aromatic oils, have a relaxing and calming effect.

Using drugs carefully

Drugs of any kind can be dangerous if used incorrectly. It is important to take any medicine exactly as recommended by the doctor or pharmacist, and never to take more than the prescribed dose. This is particularly important with painkillers, which can cause great harm if the dose is too high. Also, it is easy to become **dependent** on some types of tranquilizers.

Dependence

A serious **side effect** of some drugs, including most tranquilizers and some painkillers, is **dependence.** This is often called getting hooked or becoming addicted. A person becomes so used to the drug that they feel they must keep taking it. They might even feel they cannot live without it. The severity of the problem can vary from person to person. It is affected by the dose the individual is used to taking and the length of time he or she has been using the drug.

Physical dependence

Dependence on a drug often has two aspects—physical and **psychological.** Physical dependence occurs when the body has developed a chemical need for the drug. Without it, the body cannot continue working as before. When the drug is stopped, this has effects on the body called **withdrawal symptoms.** These can often be more unpleasant and more severe than the original problem that the drug was supposed to treat. Each type of drug creates its own range of withdrawal symptoms. These include aches and pains, muscle cramps, sweating, **nausea,** and uncontrollable shaking and crying.

Psychological dependence

Psychological dependence is based in the feelings and emotions of the mind. People believe that they must have the drug or they will not be able to cope. There may be great sensations of pleasure, well-being, and security from taking the drug, which will be shattered if the drug is stopped. The withdrawal symptoms often include **depression** and anxiety. In both physical and psychological dependence, there is a temptation to take just one more pill to ward off withdrawal symptoms. Another temptation is to take another drug in order to treat the withdrawal symptoms of the first.

Depression and lack of hope may occur both with dependence and withdrawal.

Drug tolerance

Drug **tolerance** occurs when the usual dose of the drug has less and less effect each time it is taken. To gain the same effect as before, the dose has to be increased. Tolerance can rise to a point where the amount of the drug is so high in each dose that it begins to have toxic (poisonous) effects on the body. This does not happen during normal use.

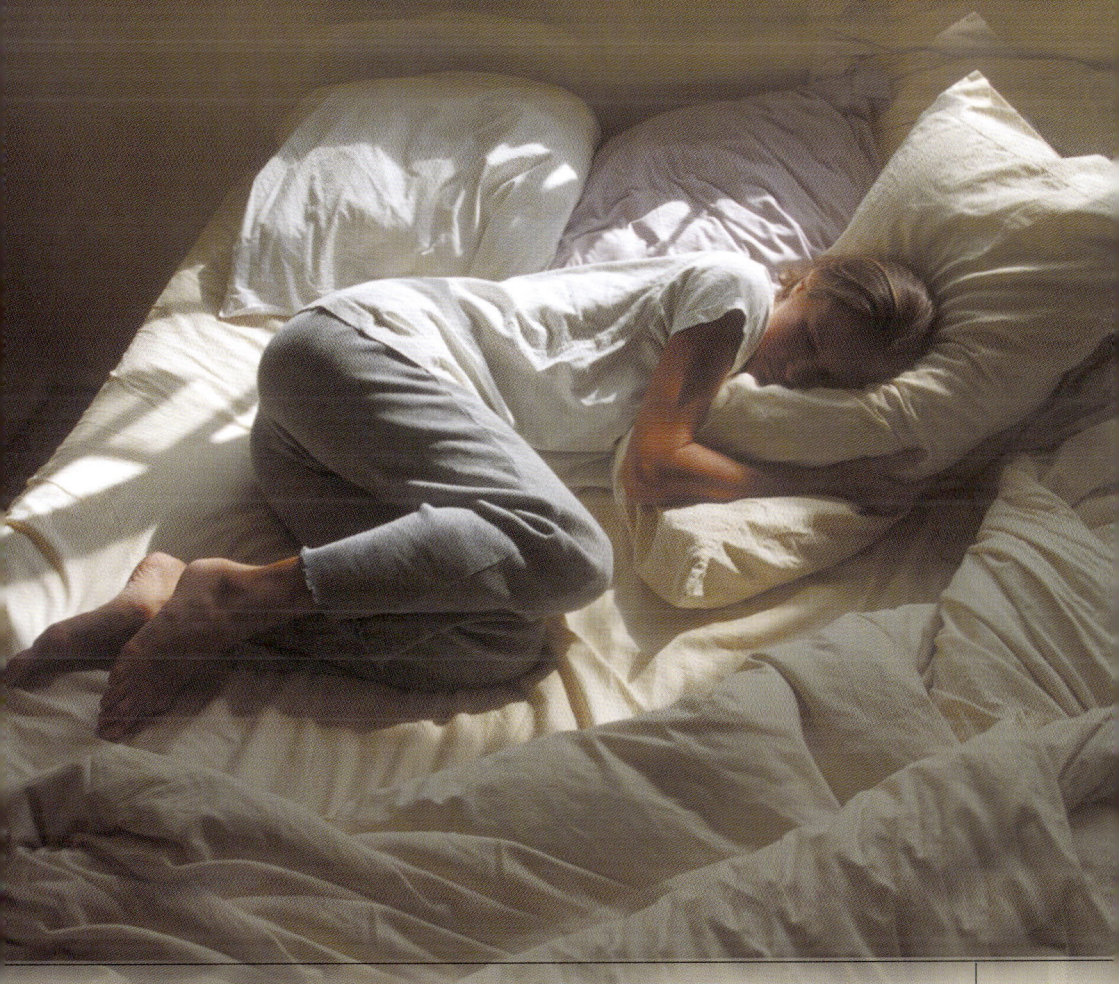

Painkiller dependence

Most **over-the-counter** painkillers carry no risk of physical **dependency.** However, some people become dependent on painkillers that contain small amounts of the more powerful opiate-based painkiller, **codeine.** In some countries, codeine is often mixed with less powerful drugs, such as **acetaminophen,** to make pills that are sold as over-the-counter painkillers.

No warnings

There is no international agreement to put warnings about dependency on the packaging of painkillers with codeine or similar drugs. An estimated 1.5 million Americans take prescription painkillers for nonmedical reasons. When they stop taking the pills, they might not understand why they feel worse.

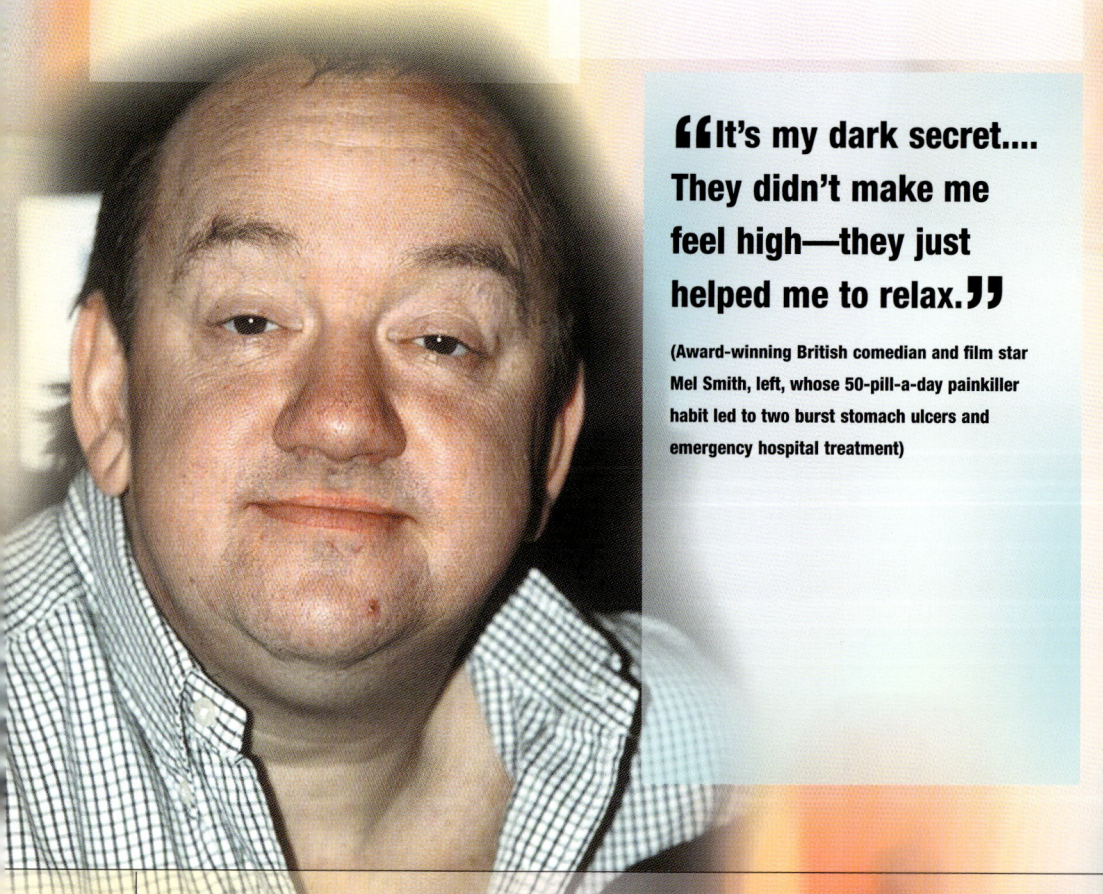

> **It's my dark secret.... They didn't make me feel high—they just helped me to relax.**
>
> (Award-winning British comedian and film star Mel Smith, left, whose 50-pill-a-day painkiller habit led to two burst stomach ulcers and emergency hospital treatment)

In a few cases, people who take very high doses of codeine-containing painkillers build up a chemical **tolerance**. This means they have to take even more, up to 70 pills a day, just to continue feeling normal. These painkillers are available only in limited quantities to reduce the danger of **overdose**.

Controlled painkillers

Powerful **opiate-opioid** painkillers can be legally used only under medical supervision, so that risks of dependence and tolerance can be assessed. If taken illegally, opiate drugs such as **heroin** and **morphine** can soon lead to both tolerance and dependence. It is possible for some people to live near-normal lives for many years while they are dependent on heroin. But hundreds die every year from accidental overdose, contaminated doses (with poisonous substances added), and infected needles and equipment. Thousands more go to prison, having turned to crime to obtain the money to pay for the drug.

Heroin withdrawal

Physical **withdrawal** from opiates-opioids such as heroin usually lasts about ten days and is likened to severe flu symptoms, including sweating, aches, pains, muscle spasms, sickness, and stomach cramps. **Psychological** dependence tends to last much longer. Ex-users often need support and counseling for months, as well as a change of surroundings and lifestyle, in order to kick the habit.

37

Tranquilizer dependence

Dependence on **benzodiazepine** tranquilizers was a huge problem in the 1980s and 1990s, and is still an issue today. About 100 million benzodiazepine prescriptions are written in the United States each year. It has been called the third great addiction, after alcohol and the drug nicotine in tobacco. People take the amount of benzodiazepine they need to keep them going, just as nicotine users smoke a certain number of cigarettes each day.

Getting hooked

It is impossible to become hooked after taking just one benzodiazepine pill. But if these tranquilizers are taken regularly, the risk of dependence rises steeply after about two months. After a year, dependence is almost certain. The affected person continues taking the same amount each day, perhaps for years. Yet the drug may have stopped working after only a few weeks. This is why benzodiazepine tranquilizers should not be taken for more than four weeks.

Recognizing dependence

Dependence on benzodiazepines is quite common, but is not always easy to recognize or understand. Doctors look for signs such as loss of alertness, poor memory, clumsiness, and, sometimes, aggressive behavior.

People who become dependent on a drug may think, "I'll just take one more, then I'll stop."

38

Withdrawal symptoms

Withdrawal symptoms caused by suddenly stopping benzodiazepines can be as varied as they are severe. They include:
- aches and pains;
- restlessness;
- irregular heartbeat;
- sweating;
- loss of appetite; and
- loss of muscle control including "the shakes."

There may also be a return to the problems that the tranquilizer was originally supposed to treat, such as anxiety, restlessness, lack of sleep, and panic attacks. It can be difficult to know if these problems are the effects of **withdrawal,** or the original symptoms coming back again.

Barbiturate dependence

Tolerance and dependence on **barbiturates** are serious problems, similar to those of hard drugs such as **heroin** or cocaine. The problems are relatively rare today because barbiturates themselves are rarely used or misused.

"Shadow world"—the story of Charles

The story of Charles shows the problems that heavy **dependence** on tranquilizers can cause. Charles was just 21 years old when he complained to his doctor that he felt tired and run-down. He felt he needed a pick-me-up. This was 1964, just as **benzodiazepine** tranquilizers were becoming popular, but before their risks were understood. The doctor prescribed tranquilizers.

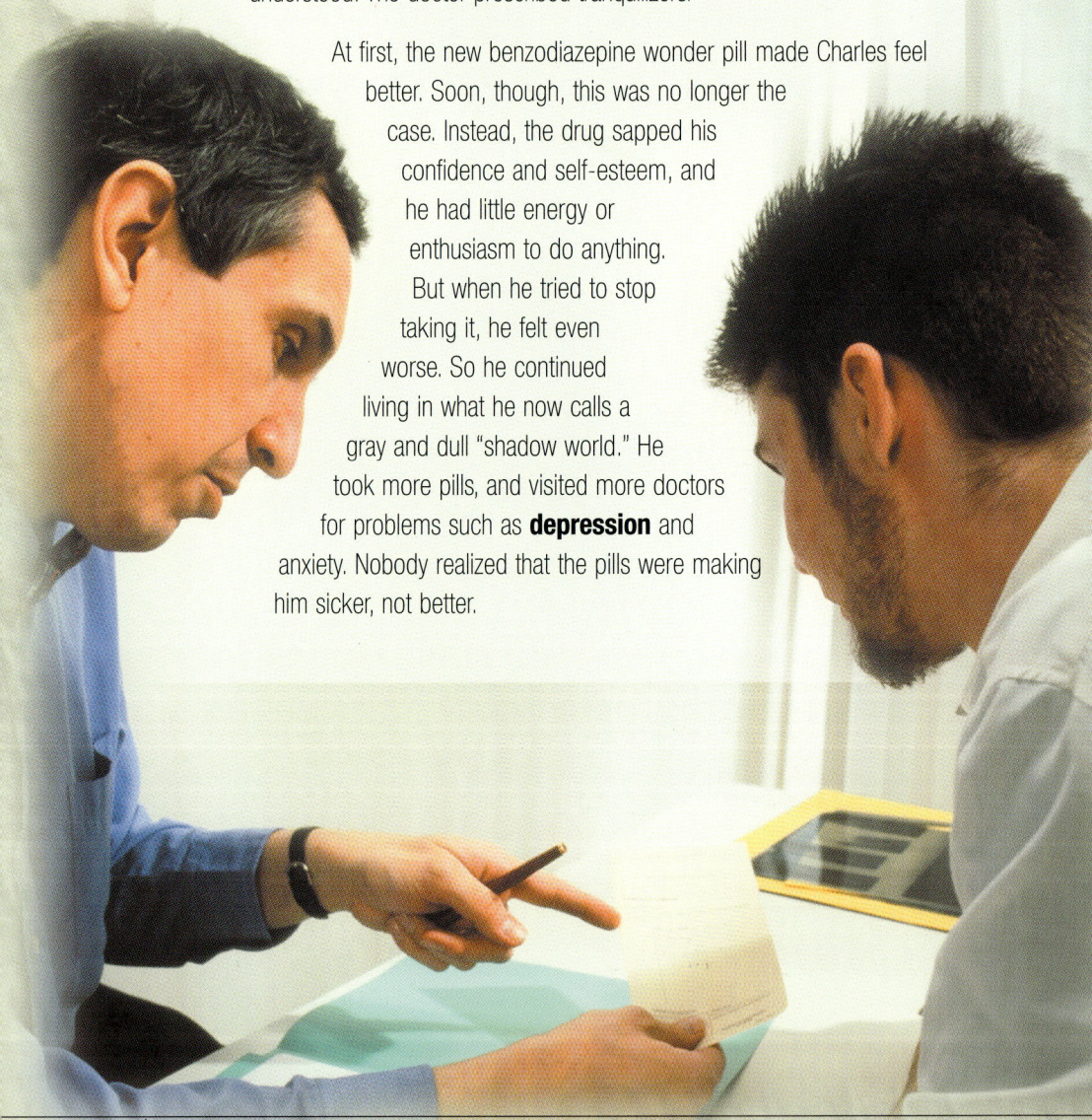

At first, the new benzodiazepine wonder pill made Charles feel better. Soon, though, this was no longer the case. Instead, the drug sapped his confidence and self-esteem, and he had little energy or enthusiasm to do anything. But when he tried to stop taking it, he felt even worse. So he continued living in what he now calls a gray and dull "shadow world." He took more pills, and visited more doctors for problems such as **depression** and anxiety. Nobody realized that the pills were making him sicker, not better.

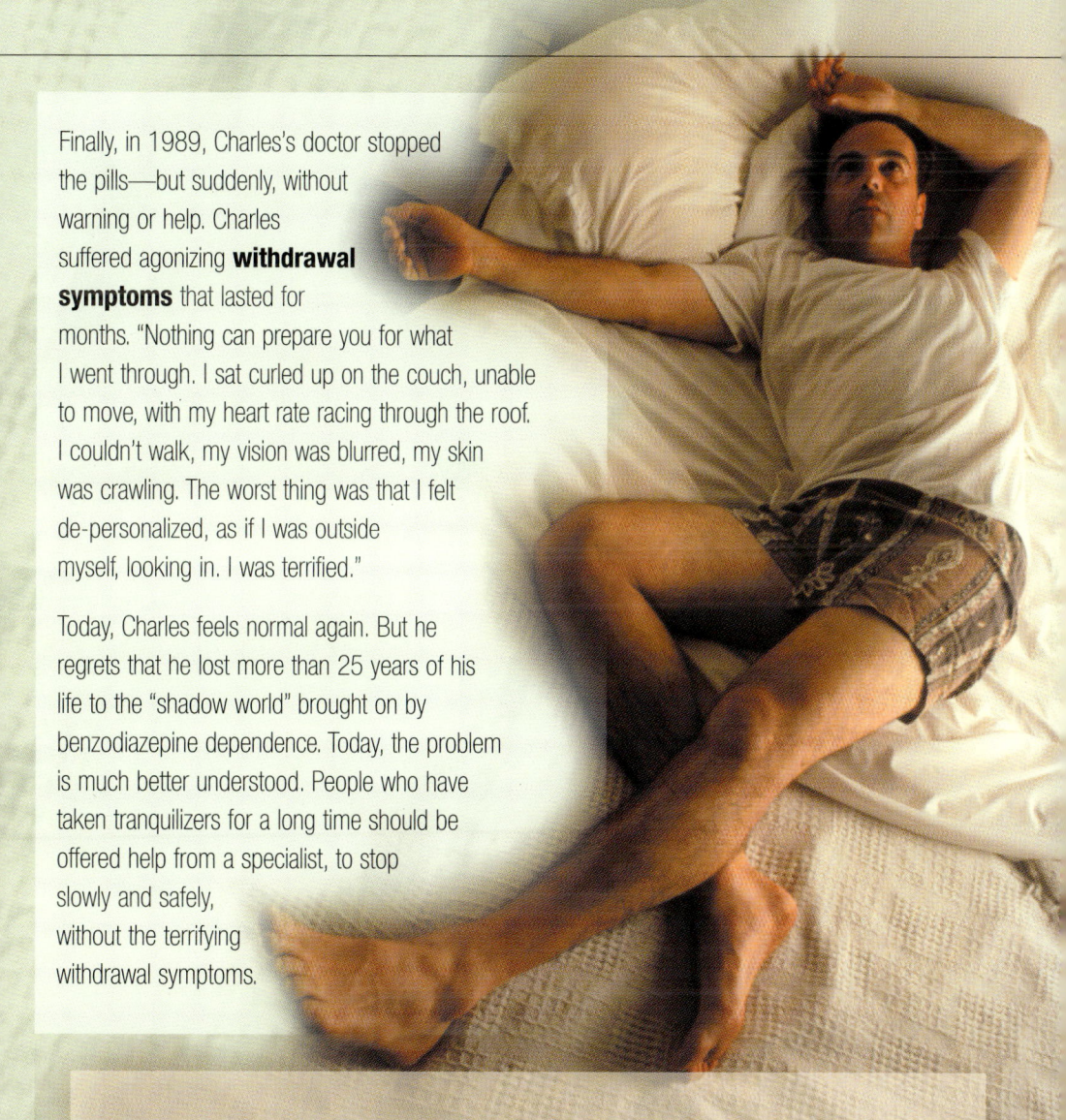

Finally, in 1989, Charles's doctor stopped the pills—but suddenly, without warning or help. Charles suffered agonizing **withdrawal symptoms** that lasted for months. "Nothing can prepare you for what I went through. I sat curled up on the couch, unable to move, with my heart rate racing through the roof. I couldn't walk, my vision was blurred, my skin was crawling. The worst thing was that I felt de-personalized, as if I was outside myself, looking in. I was terrified."

Today, Charles feels normal again. But he regrets that he lost more than 25 years of his life to the "shadow world" brought on by benzodiazepine dependence. Today, the problem is much better understood. People who have taken tranquilizers for a long time should be offered help from a specialist, to stop slowly and safely, without the terrifying withdrawal symptoms.

"At that time benzodiazepine was regarded as a panacea, a cure-all. I was told it would get me back on my feet. Nobody warned me about any side effects. What I really needed was a break, like a vacation. Instead, I ended up becoming an addict."

(Charles today)

Stopping Tranquilizers

There are no set rules about **dependence** on tranquilizers or other drugs, or about their **side effects** or **withdrawal symptoms.** Each person reacts differently. In general, people who have been prescribed **benzodiazepine** tranquilizers for more than a month should seriously question both themselves and the doctor about why these drugs are still needed. The longer someone uses benzodiazepines, the greater the dependence. It becomes much more difficult to stop using the drug, and the withdrawal symptoms become much worse.

A vicious cycle

The first sign of trouble is often a feeling that the benzodiazepine drug is not working like it should. Indeed, this is probably true, since the body has gotten used to it and developed a **tolerance.** Some of the original symptoms, such as anxiety and worry, difficulty in sleeping, and restlessness, might return. In addition, the person is likely to experience new feelings of irritability and tension. It may seem that the way to feel better is to take more of the drug. But this means tolerance and dependence increase, too. When this happens, the patient has entered a spiral of dependence, or a vicious cycle.

The decision to stop

If this happens, the patient has to make some clear decisions, with the aid of a doctor and especially with a tranquilizer-dependency counselor or someone else experienced in such problems. The patient must be certain that he or she wants to get off the drug, because their life in the long term will be better without it. Once that decision has been made, the patient needs to follow a series of carefully planned steps.

Stopping benzodiazepines

To suddenly stop taking a benzodiazepine tranquilizer, after taking one regularly, can cause enormous problems. When the body is abruptly deprived of the drug, after months or years of use, the withdrawal symptoms can be extremely serious. They include severe confusion, **convulsions, hallucinations,** and many other dangerous effects. Even for patients who have been taking the drug for only a short time, stopping suddenly can bring on rebound anxiety. The feelings of worry and agitation are far worse than they originally were when the patient started taking tranquilizers.

Withdrawal symptoms for benzodiazepines include confusion, strange feelings, fearful thoughts, and great agitation.

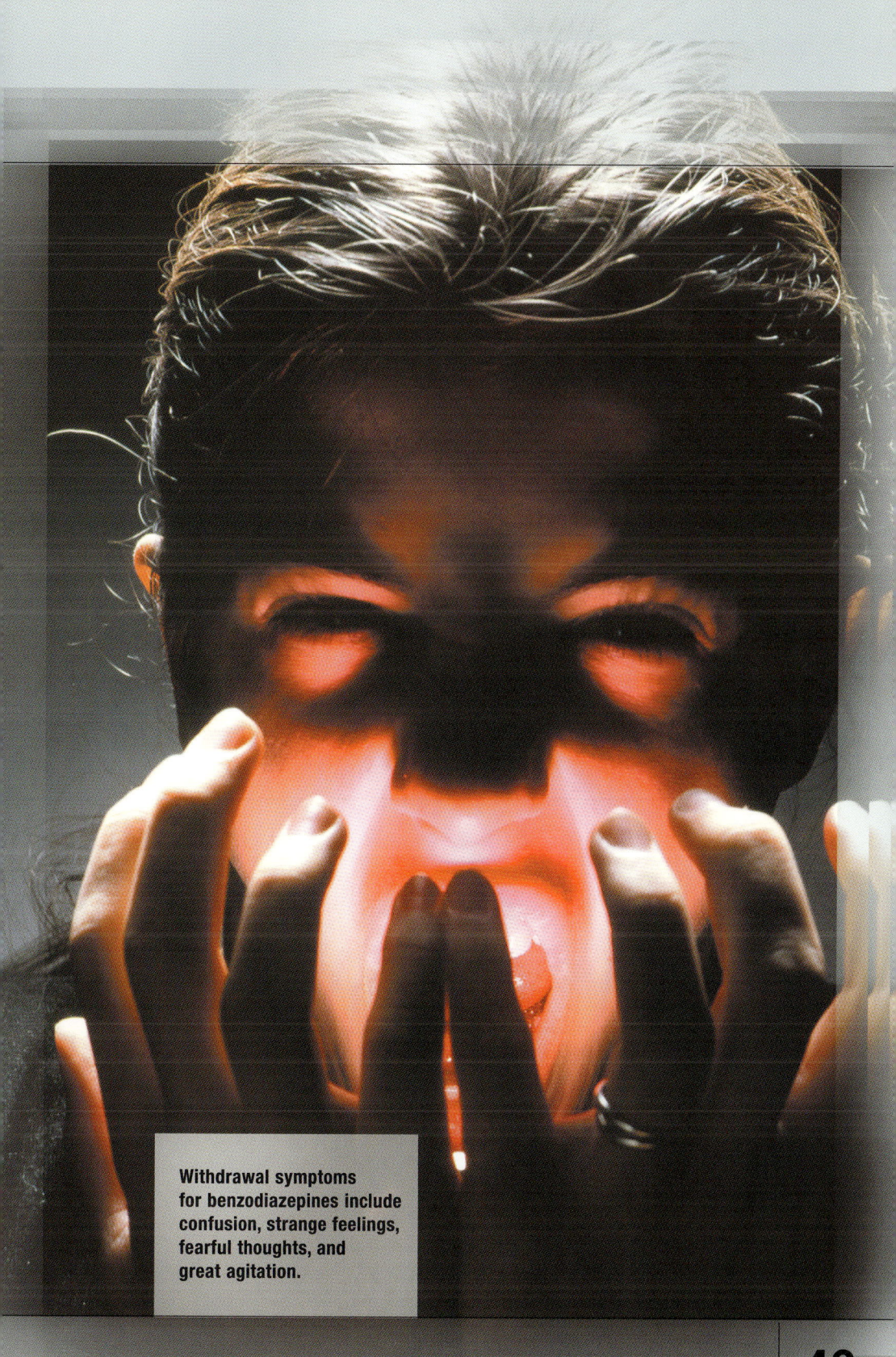

Anyone can stop taking **benzodiazepine** tranquilizers. But nobody who is **dependent** on them can expect to quit overnight. **Withdrawal** from a benzodiazepine tranquilizer must be done very slowly and carefully.

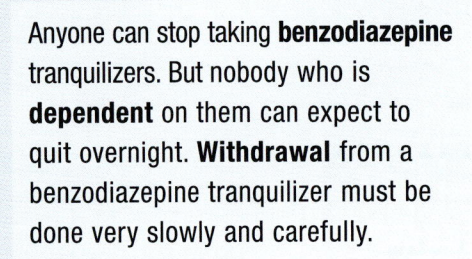

Reducing the dose

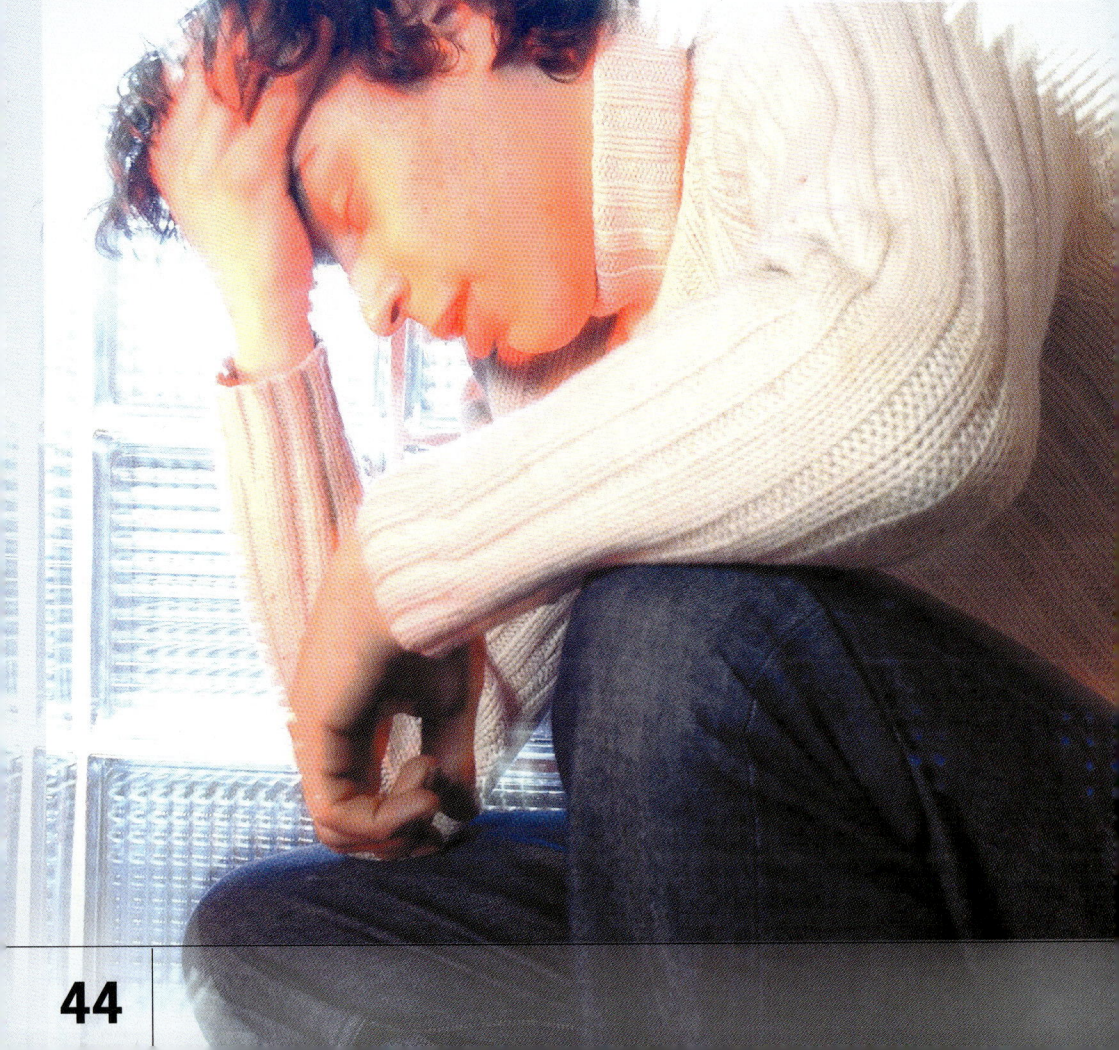

The main goal is to gradually reduce, over a period of weeks or even months, the amount of benzodiazepine tranquilizer taken. This is called **tapering** the dose of the drug. In one form of tapering withdrawal program, the total daily dose of benzodiazepine is reduced by roughly one-eighth. This reduced dose is kept constant as it is taken each day for two to three weeks. Then it is reduced again, by one-eighth of its new total, and taken for another two to three weeks, and so on.

Managing withdrawal

This form of withdrawal should be done with the help of a doctor and preferably an expert counselor or advisor on benzodiazepine dependency. Some patients manage the program mainly by themselves, with background medical supervision. Others need plenty of advice and support. In general, the longer a patient has taken the drug, the more gradual the withdrawal should be. This also applies to people who have taken a benzodiazepine tranquilizer for another medical reason other than anxiety, such as epilepsy.

Even during a very gradual tapering, some patients with severe tranquilizer dependence can suffer **withdrawal symptoms.** If the drug is stopped too quickly, these symptoms can include headaches, dizziness, **nausea, depression,** aching muscles, burning skin, and even **hallucinations.**

Successful withdrawal

The speed and success of the withdrawal program varies greatly. It depends on the types of drug that the person has been taking, and for how long, and how seriously dependent he or she has become. As a general guide, it usually takes at least twelve weeks for a mildly dependent user to stop. A severely dependent long-term user will need over a year. The process of clearing a tranquilizer (or other drug) from the body is called **detoxification.** When it is complete, the person can expect to return to how he or she was before ever taking the drug.

"Will my hands ever stop shaking like I have a terrible hangover? Will my brain be quiet, will my body be still, will I be able to say 'I'm happy to be alive' again? Will I believe life is worth living like I used to?"

(Jen, recovering from a benzodiazepine dependency, four months after quitting)

Alternatives to Drugs

There are many ways to cope with pain and anxiety that do not involve drugs. As with any health problem, it is important to identify the basic cause first, and deal with that if possible. For example, a person with back pain could be sitting at a desk in a bad position or lifting heavy loads using the wrong method. A person who is very nervous and restless might be having problems at school or feeling crowded and cramped by family members at home. There are endless similar examples of how to solve the cause, rather than masking the symptoms with drugs. There are also approaches using therapies, such as **psychotherapy.**

Natural remedies

Many modern drugs have been developed from traditional natural remedies. Health stores and alternative medicine suppliers stock a range of creams, pills, and lotions based on natural ingredients and plant extracts for easing pain and calming anxiety. However, these remedies sometimes react with either prescribed or **over-the-counter** drugs. Not all are safe and effective in all cases. A pharmacist or qualified expert such as a herbalist can give advice.

Yoga, a relaxation technique for mind and body, is widely used to help people cope with the stress of modern life.

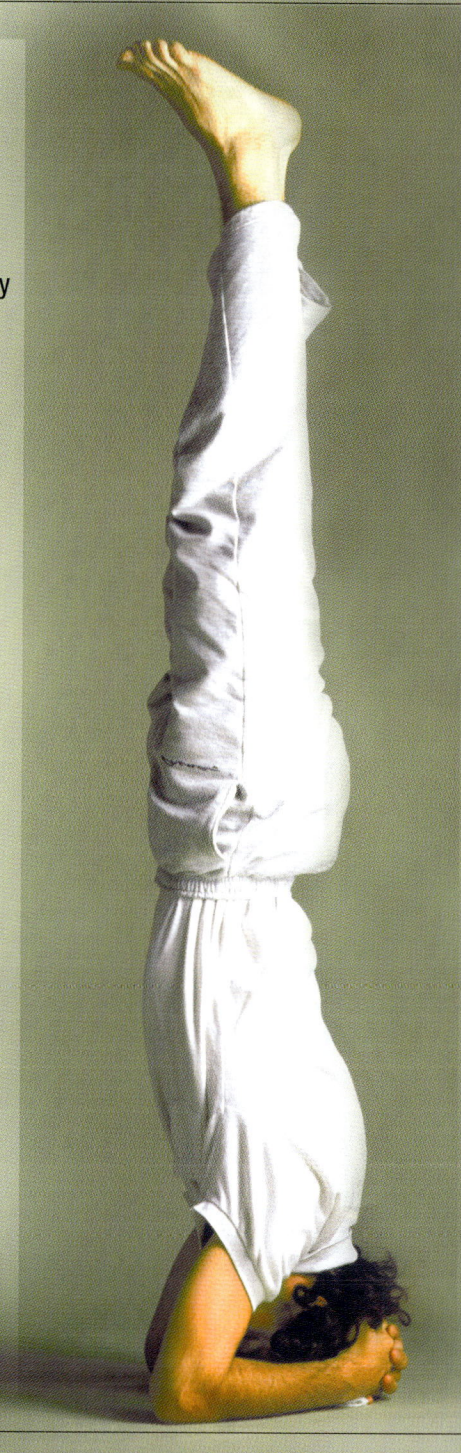

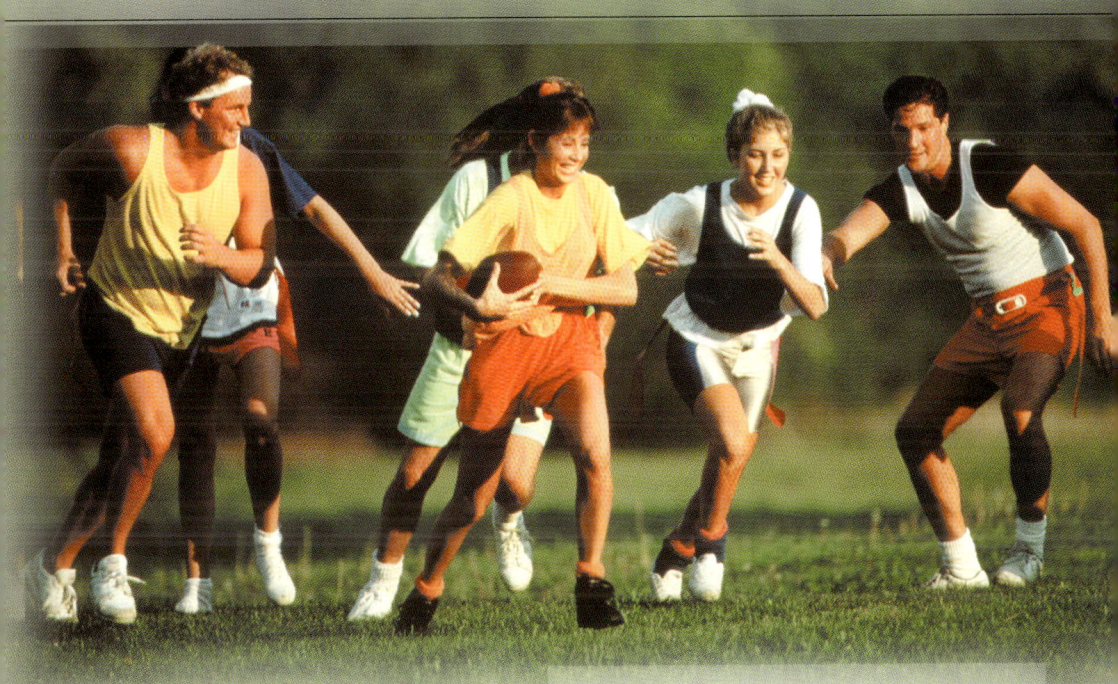

Enjoying sports and exercise, especially with other people, can be a successful way to reduce anxiety and tension.

Complementary therapy

Complementary medicines can be used in addition to **conventional medicine.** If the source of a pain is physical, such as poor posture, then a physical therapy such as manipulation, **osteopathy, chiropractic,** or **Alexander Technique** may help. One of the most ancient therapies for relief of pain and anxiety is **acupuncture.** Yoga, meditation, and **hypnotherapy** are other recognized techniques for relieving stress, anxiety, and worry.

A healthy body

Another way to maintain a healthy and positive mind and reduce anxiety is to maintain a fit, healthy body. The best way is through regular exercise, such as swimming, cycling, jogging, brisk walking, or playing sports. Exercise and physical activity release natural body chemicals called **endorphins** in the brain. Endorphins have a role as the body's natural painkillers and they also increase feelings of well-being.

Legal Matters

Tranquilizers and stronger painkillers are classed as **controlled drugs** in the United States, the United Kingdom, Australia, and many other countries. It is against the law to possess these substances without a doctor's prescription. It is illegal to possess some types at all. The penalties are severe for those who are caught.

Possession of controlled drugs without a prescription can lead to arrest.

Controlling drug use

In the United States, powers for controlling drug use are provided by the Pure Food, Drug, and Cosmetic Act (1938, plus amendments) and the Controlled Substances Act (1970). Originally, the Pure Food, Drug, and Cosmetic Act simply required the manufacturer to show that a drug was safe before it was marketed. In 1962, the act was amended to require that any drug also be proven effective, not just safe, before it was marketed. The Controlled Substances Act set up federal funds for drug education and prevention programs, classified drugs according to their medical use and abuse potential, and established legal guidelines for possessing, making, or distributing drugs.

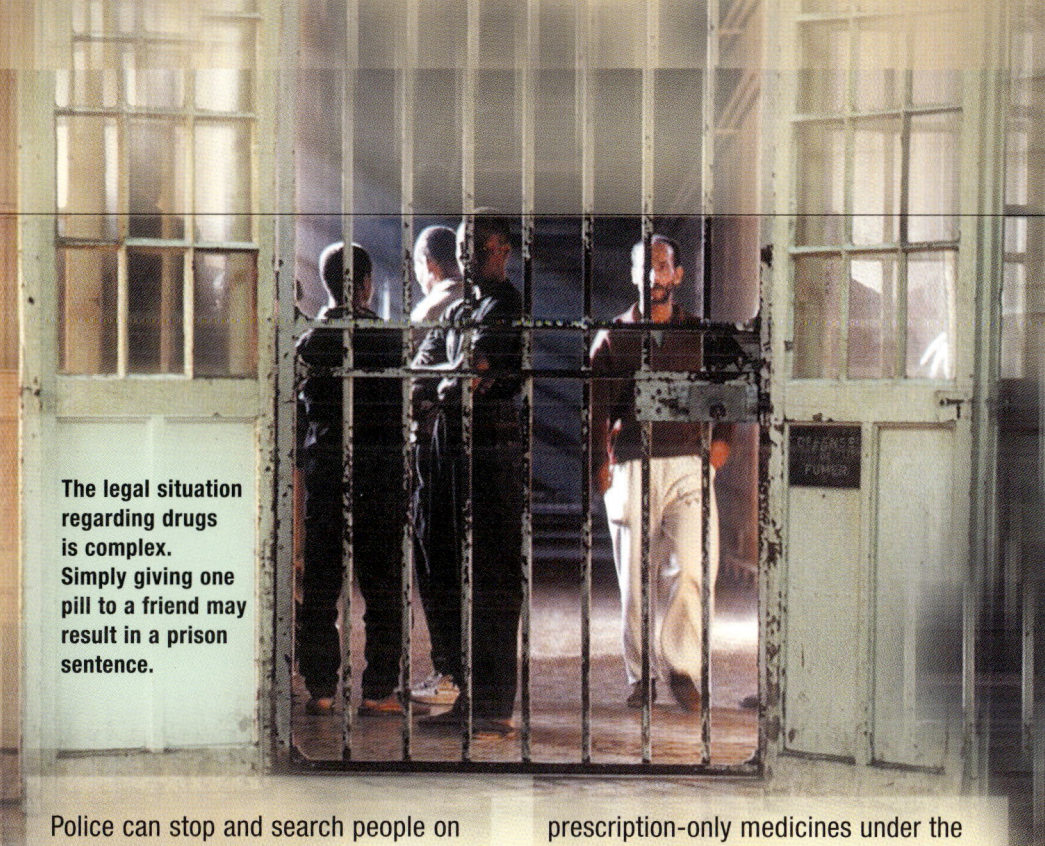

The legal situation regarding drugs is complex. Simply giving one pill to a friend may result in a prison sentence.

Police can stop and search people on reasonable suspicion that they possess a controlled drug.

In addition to these national laws, many schools, colleges, and similar organizations have their own sets of rules. These often prevent the possession, use, or sale of painkillers and other drugs on the premises. In some cases, even look-alike pills are included (they look like real drugs, but do not contain active ingredients). It is part of the drive toward safer, drug-free surroundings.

Minor tranquilizers

All minor tranquilizers, including the **benzodiazepine** group, are prescription-only medicines under the laws in the United States, United Kingdom, Australia and many other countries. This means that they can be legally supplied by prescription only.

It is illegal to supply benzodiazepines to another person. Penalties for doing so can include fines or even prison. If a person obtains tranquilizers with a doctor's prescription and sells or gives some to another person, then he or she is committing a criminal offense. For some tranquilizers, such as **temazepam** or flunitrazepam (Rohypnol), the controls are much stricter. Simply possessing them without a prescription is a serious offense. Similar strict controls and severe penalties apply to **barbiturate** tranquilizers.

49

People Who Can Help

Despite many changes in prescription guidelines and publicity campaigns, **dependence** on **benzodiazepine** tranquilizers is still a relatively common problem today. An estimated four million people in the United States have used prescribed benzodiazepines regularly for five years or more. A benzodiazepine-dependent person is advised to approach one of the official agencies or self-help groups for advice. Another starting point is to seek help more informally from a family member, a trusted friend, a member of a church or reputable religious group, or a trained counselor. It is valuable to talk, listen, and take advice. The next stage is to find expert help for guidance and support through the **withdrawal** process.

Self-help groups

Self-help groups for tranquilizer dependency exist in many countries. People can meet, share their concerns, and get advice by phone or over the Internet. Often the groups are run by people who have had experience with being dependent on benzodiazepines themselves. Similar groups also offer help for problems with dependency on common **over-the-counter** painkillers.

Starting points for beating benzodiazepine dependency

These sources can provide information on local self-help groups, usually free of charge. Generally, the group members remain anonymous.
- family doctor
- local health or medical center
- local library information lists
- trained counselor in health and medical matters
- community center
- drug treatment services, substance abuse centers, or **detoxification** centers, listed in phone books, libraries, and on the Internet

Most national organizations offer free advice over the phone, put people in touch with expert help, supply brochures and videos, and possibly arrange home visits.

Self-help sessions allow people to realize they are not alone, share their experiences, and receive first-hand advice about coping with drug dependence and withdrawal.

Future directions

Drug companies spend billions of dollars each year on researching new products, including new types of tranquilizers and painkillers. In many cases, tranquilizers are gradually being phased out and replaced by **antidepressants.** Research into new painkillers includes the development of drugs such as Cox-2 inhibitors. They also have anti-cancer effects, but in tests some types have been shown to affect the digestive system, the liver, and the healing of wounds. Marijuana, which is currently an illegal drug, also has pain-relieving effects. Research is being carried out to determine whether the substances in it that have these effects can be made into safe prescription drugs.

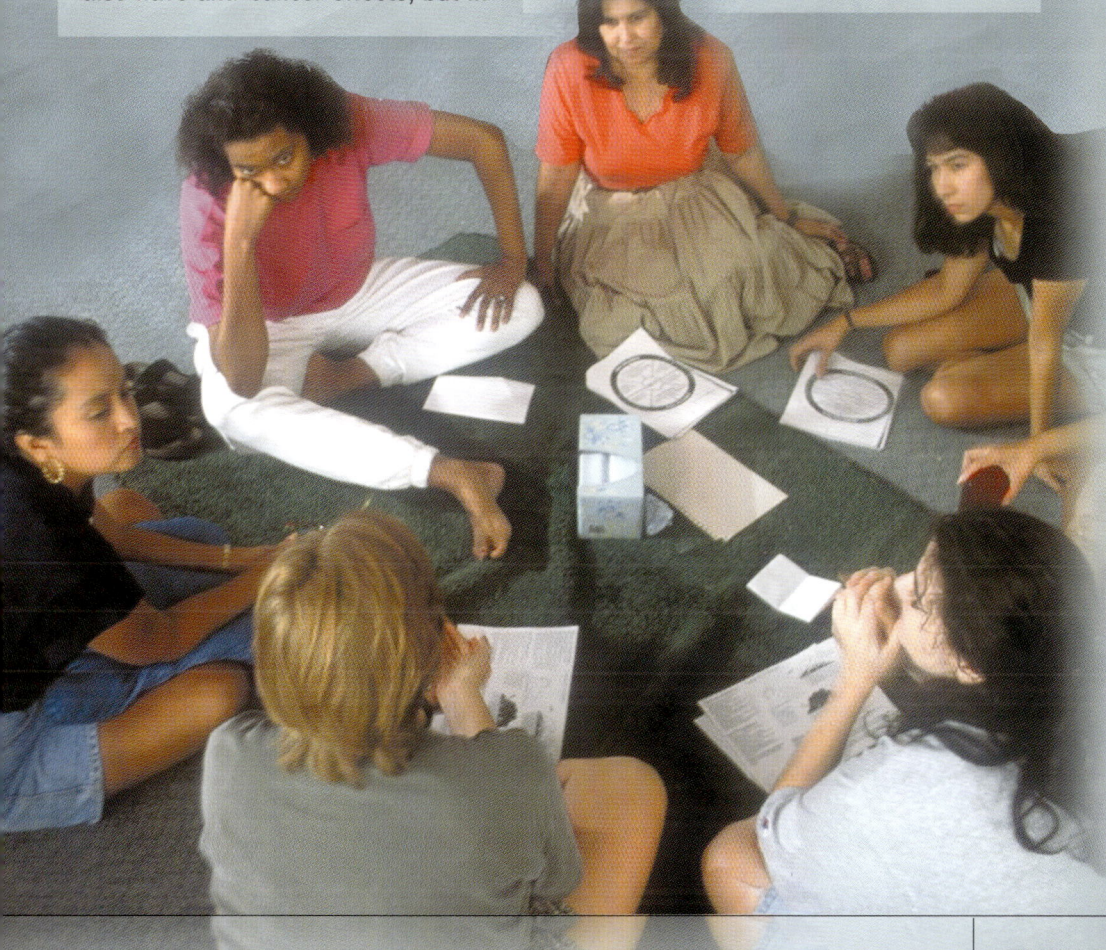

51

Information and Advice

Many organizations and groups offer general information about drugs and how to cope with pain, anxiety, and **depression.** Some organizations offer specific help with **withdrawal** from tranquilizers and **over-the-counter** painkillers. Contacts listed here can also provide information on organizations that provide help to cope with painful medical conditions such as back pain, arthritis, and cancer.

Contacts

American Pain Society
4700 W. Lake Avenue
Glenview, IL 60025
(847) 375-4715
http://www.ampainsoc.org
This organization aims to advance pain-related research, education, treatment, and professional practice.

Center for Substance Abuse Prevention (CSAP)
1010 Wayne Avenue, Suite 850
Silver Spring, MD 20910
(301) 459-1591, ext. 244
http://www.covesoft.com/csap.html
CSAP is a federal program that provides information and helps communities to combat alcohol and drug problems.

Drug Abuse Resistance Education (D.A.R.E.)
P.O. Box 512090
Los Angeles, CA 90051
(800) 223-3273
http://www.dare.com
D.A.R.E. is a national organization that links law-enforcement and educational resources to provide up-to-date and comprehensive information about all aspects of drug use.

National Chronic Pain Outreach Association
P.O. Box 274
Millboro, VA 24460
(540) 862-9437
This nonprofit organization offers a wide range of publications and audio tapes relating to pain.

National Institute on Drug Abuse (NIDA)
6001 Executive Blvd., Room 5213
Bethesda, MD 20892
(301) 443-1124
http://www.nida.nih.gov/
NIDA works to improve drug abuse and addiction prevention treatment and policy. They also have information on drug abuse for students, parents, teachers, and health professionals.

National Pain Foundation
P.O. Box 102605
Denver, CO 80250
(303) 756-0889
http://www.painconnection.org
This is a nonprofit organization that provides online information for pain patients and their families. They have information on pain, treatment options, and support groups.

More Books to Read

Connolly, Sean. *Heroin.* Chicago: Heinemann Library, 2001.

Grabish, Beatrice R. *Drugs and Your Brain.* New York: Rosen Publishing Group, Inc., 1998.

Jaffe, Steven L. (ed.) *How to Get Help.* Broomall, Penn.: Chelsea House, 1999.

Masline, Shelagh Ryan. *Drug Abuse and Teens.* Berkeley Heights, N.J.: Enslow Publishers, Inc., 2000.

Moe, Barbara. *Drug Abuse Relapse: Helping Teens to Get Clean Again.* New York: Rosen Publishing Group, Inc., 2000.

Myers, Arthur. *Drugs and Emotions.* New York: Rosen Publishing Group, Inc., 1996.

Roberts, Jeremy. *Prescription Drug Abuse.* New York: Rosen Publishing Group, Inc., 2000.

Torr, James D. and Scott Barbour. *Drug Abuse.* San Diego, Calif.: Greenhaven Press, Inc., 1999.

Wallerstein, Claire. *Depression.* Chicago: Heinemann Library, 2003.

Westcott, Patsy. *Why Do People Take Drugs?* Chicago: Raintree Publishers, 2001.

Disclaimer
All the Internet addresses (URLs) given in this book were valid at the time of going to press. However, due to the dynamic nature of the Internet, some addresses may have changed, or sites may have changed or ceased to exist since publication. While the authors and publisher regret any inconvenience this may cause readers, no responsibility for any such changes can be accepted by either the authors or the publisher.

Glossary

acetaminophen widely-used drug to relieve aches and pains, usually safe for babies and young people, but very dangerous in overdose

acupuncture ancient Eastern technique of pain relief and treatment for well-being, usually using needles placed into the skin

Alexander Technique technique using posture and exercise to relieve illness and promote well-being

anesthetic substance that causes reduction or loss in sensation or feeling, including pain

analgesic substance that lessens or reduces pain

antidepressant drug prescribed by doctors to treat depression

anti-inflammatory substance that reduces swelling and pain

anxiolytic substance that relieves anxiety

aspirin widely-used drug to relieve aches, pains, stiffness, and inflammation

barbiturate powerful tranquilizer rarely used today

benzodiazepine type of tranquilizer or antianxiety drug, also used to treat sleeplessness

chiropractic treatment in which the spine is adjusted to help cure health problems

codeine pain-relieving drug with high dependence risk

complementary therapy therapy used in conjunction with conventional medicine to treat aspects of an illness that conventional medicine may not be able to deal with easily

controlled drug substance that is subject to laws, regulations, or legal restrictions

conventional medicine medicine practiced by most doctors and hospitals in the Western world

convulsion fit or seizure; when the body makes uncontrolled, often jerky movements

dependence continuing need or desire for a substance, even when it no longer works

depression feelings of extreme sadness, hopelessness, and lack of energy

detoxification ridding the body of a harmful or toxic substance

endorphin natural substance in the body that acts in the nervous system and brain to reduce feelings of pain

hallucination something that seems real but is not, and is solely in the mind, including sights, sounds, smells, tastes, skin sensations, and pain

heroin powerful narcotic drug that relieves pain; it has many side effects and a high risk of dependency

hypnotherapy treatment that includes sending a patient into a state of deep relaxation in which he or she can still see and hear and follow commands

hypnotic substance that brings on feelings of drowsiness or altered consciousness; *see also* narcotic

ibuprofen widely-used drug to relieve aches, pains, stiffness, and inflammation

Librium brand name for chlordiazepoxide, a benzodiazepine tranquilizer or antianxiety drug

Mogadon brand name for nitrazepam, a benzodiazepine tranquilizer or antianxiety drug used as a sleeping pill

morphine powerful narcotic drug that relieves pain; it also has many side effects and a high risk of dependency

narcotic substance that brings on feelings of drowsiness or altered consciousness, and that may have risks of dependence; *see also* hypnotic

nausea feeling of being sick or about to throw up

nervous breakdown common but misleading term for a time when a person cannot cope with daily life, due to an underlying problem such as a mental illness

NSAID non-steroidal anti-inflammatory drug; can be painkillers such as aspirin, ibuprofen, and many others

opiate-opioid collective name for powerful narcotic drugs with a chemical make-up similar to substances such as morphine, originally derived from the opium poppy

opium substance derived from the sweet sap of certain poppy plants, containing various substances that act as powerful narcotic drugs

osteopathy treatment of illness and pain by pressing and moving the bones and muscles

over-the-counter (OTC) drug substance that can be bought without a doctor's prescription

overdose act of taking too much of a substance into the body, so that it has harmful or even deadly effects

psychological having to do with human behavior, the mind, and mental activities

psychotherapy treatment used for problems based in the mind rather than the physical body

recreational user person who uses drugs or substances occasionally, for nonmedical purposes

sedative having a soothing, calming, or tranquilizing effect

side effect change caused by a drug in the mind or body that is not the intended effect and which may be harmful

tapering to gradually reduce the dose of a drug

temazepam benzodiazepine tranquilizer or antianxiety drug used as a sleeping pill

tolerance when the same amount of a drug gradually has less and less effect, so more and more of it is needed to maintain the original effect

Valium brand name for diazepam, a benzodiazepine tranquilizer or antianxiety drug

withdrawal act or process of discontinuing a drug

withdrawal symptom effect, usually unpleasant, that occurs when a drug is no longer taken; symptoms may include sweating, muscle spasms, pain, sickness, and hallucinations

Index

A acetaminophen 6, 16, 17, 18, 36, 55
addiction 29, 34, 38, 41
alcohol 5, 10, 23
    pain relief 8
    recreational drugs 31
Alexander Technique 47, 54
analgesics 6, 16, 54
anesthetics 9, 54
anti-inflammatory drugs 14, 16
antidepressants 27, 28–29, 51, 54
anxiolytics 25, 54
aspirin 6, 9, 14, 16, 17, 54
    side effects 18, 19

B barbiturates 25, 39, 49, 54
benzodiazepines 10, 11, 24–25, 54
    controlled drugs 49
    dependence 38, 40, 41, 42, 50
    prescription drugs 33
    recreational use 31
    side effects 26–27
    withdrawal 42, 43, 44, 45
brain 12, 14, 19, 25

C cocaine 39
codeine 17, 36, 37, 54
complementary therapies 5, 33, 47, 54
controlled drugs 6, 48–49, 54

D dependence 5, 30, 33, 34–39, 40, 54
    barbiturates 25, 39
    help 50
    opiate-opioids 6, 16, 36, 37
    painkillers 34, 36, 37
    tranquilizers 11, 30, 33, 34, 38, 40–41, 42, 44, 45
depression 21, 27, 29, 34, 40, 45, 52, 54
detoxification 45, 54

E endorphins 47, 54

H hallucinations 42, 45, 54
heroin 6, 16, 17, 39, 55
    dependence 25, 37
    recreational use 30, 31
hypnotherapy 33, 47, 54

I ibuprofen 14, 16, 17, 18, 19, 54
illegal drug trade 5, 23

L laudanum 8
laws 48–49
Librium 10, 11, 22, 25, 55

M marijuana 51
Mogadon 10, 24, 31, 55
morphine 6, 16, 17, 37, 55

N narcotics 16, 55
natural remedies 8, 10, 46
NSAIDs 16, 19, 55

O opiate-opioids 6, 16, 30, 31, 36, 37, 55
opium 6, 8, 10, 55
over-the-counter drugs 19, 46, 50, 52, 55
    opiates 17
    painkillers 5, 16, 32, 36
overdose 5, 55
    acetaminophen 16, 19
    barbiturates 25
    natural medicines 8
    painkillers 37

P pethidine 16, 17
prescribed drugs 46, 48, 49, 50, 51
    painkillers 5, 6, 36
    tranquilizers 5, 6, 32, 38
psychotherapy 33, 46, 55

R recreational drug use 30, 48, 55

S sedatives 6, 10, 26, 28, 55
side effects 5, 8, 34
    acetaminophen 16
    analgesics 6
    barbiturates 25
    benzodiazepine 41
    opiates 6
    painkillers 18–19, 32
    tranquilizers 26–27, 42
sleeping difficulties 6, 20, 33, 42
    narcotics 16
    natural remedies 10
sleeping pills 25
street drugs 30–31

T temazepam 24, 31, 49, 55
tolerance 25, 35, 37, 39, 42, 55

V Valium 10, 25, 31, 55

W withdrawal 44, 45, 50, 52, 55
withdrawal symptoms 34, 55
    barbiturates 25
    benzodiazepines 39, 41
    opiates 37
    tranquilizers 42, 43, 45